WHAT READERS SAY...

"This Resource Guide is an absolute must if you want to save multiple thousands in costs. If you want to also have more time to provide a higher level of care to your loved one(s), then this Resource Guide is for you! Dr. Superson captured all the lessons I learned taking care of my own parents and opened my eyes to all the opportunities I missed during that time. Now in my 70s, my wife and I are using this Resource Guide to plan and prepare for our own future—to avoid all the needless costs in time and money I experienced. I do not wish to pass on those stressful times to my own children. The information is short, sweet, and to the point. I love it! Highly recommend!"
Paul J. Dronka—Retired Col. (U.S. Army)
Texas

"With a disabled daughter, this book has been a lifesaver! All the legwork is done for you, and the money and time saved not having to do all the research myself has been invaluable!"
Donna Lassetter
Nevada

"This Resource Guide is nothing short of a gift from God. Dealing with the heart-aching, time-consuming process of caring for someone who can't care for themselves, is difficult and stressful enough. Knowing there are so many valuable free resources out there to help makes it so much easier to deal with—and this book provides it all!"
David T. Fagan—DavidTFagan.com & former CEO Guerilla Marketing
California

"Resources are few, and help appears nonexistent—at least that's the way it feels. The fact is, there are many resources available for caregivers and for those being cared for, if only we knew about them. I wish *Essential Resource Guide for Caregivers* had been around when I cared for my dad in his final months. Both his life and mine would have been so much better. Patients often outlive their caregivers due to the heavy physical, mental, and emotional toll—and this book is a must-have for anyone who is a caregiver or is about to enter into that role.
Make *sure* a copy of this book is on hand!"
Rick Allen
Arizona

"This book is an amazing resource, and has allowed me as a social worker, to better service those in need. The tips on food stamps and free food availability helped six (6) families I personally know—which made a difference to ensure their families have access to food."
Leah Williamson—Social Worker
Tennessee

"Being a caregiver and owner of an assisted living home, the sections of this Resource Guide related to dealing with government agencies, seeking affordable and free healthy food, vision care, clothing, as well as handling the hardest part of caregiving—the financial aspects—has been invaluable and extremely helpful.

It is indeed the resource everyone should be reading—as sooner or later, almost everyone will need many of the resources found in this book. A *must own* for everyone!"

Ethel Luzario
Arizona

"This book has been a helpful guide in searching for benefits for my family. The book is loaded with information on government programs we learned we qualified for. Along with many services I found we could use, I discovered I had free burial benefits due to my military service. The information is well organized and easy to understand. Web addresses and contact information are provided so you are able to apply or obtain information quickly and easily. Thank you Dr. Superson for taking the time to put this book together. It has helped my family immensely!"

Tony Aimonetti—Veteran (U.S. Air Force)
Arizona

"*Essential Resource Guide for Caregivers* is an invaluable resource. I wish it was available when my sister and I were caregivers to our ailing aunt and uncle, as it could have saved thousands of dollars and valuable time needlessly lost searching for information.

We have already been able to utilize several of the resources ourselves and have shared it with friends who were able to take immediate advantage of all the amazing information available.

Everything is so easy to access!"

Sue Kreuter
Illinois

"As a school counselor and community advocate, *Essential Resource Guide for Caregivers* is an indispensable resource that empowers caregivers and service professionals. In a world of broken systems, the information provided goes beyond the basics and provides access to so many free, untapped, and needed resources—in a currency of loving service. I highly recommend!"

Laura Marcos—Intuitive Educator / Alchemy for Everyone
Arizona

"My mom has advanced Parkinson's disease and even though she has many children to help—the resources in this book are invaluable. Being able to have the phone numbers and websites to the companies at my fingertips was so helpful. I love the chapter on financials. This area often gets overlooked, and leaves families dealing with a lot of challenges. The chapter I also loved was about emotional care. We all have to realize how draining it is on a caregiver and need to remember they also need to be at their best to care for someone else. A MUST read!"

Holly Porter—HollyPorter.com
Utah

"I found Dr. Superson's book very helpful in navigating a system that is not set up to easily and automatically help the disabled. This book is a *must* read!"
Tamara Linnan
Arizona

"This book is the best resource on the market today. Years of research and thought have gone into putting this resource guide together for caregivers or anyone in need of basic necessities or programs—including those that are free. There is no excuse anymore to go without, if you just know where to look for these resources. Camille tells you exactly where they are located and how to access them. That is why I've had her on my radio show 4 (four) times—more than any other guest I've ever interviewed. Thank you, Camille!"
Dave Nassaney—The Caregiver's Caregiver/ "Caregiver Dave Show" / CaregiverDave.com
California

"*Essential Resource Guide for Caregivers* is nothing short of genius. It has become an important resource for those I serve. I can't say enough about the valuable information this book contains to help caregivers and their families."
Tamera Hunter—Executive Director & Co-founder of Chemo Buddies 4Life (cb4l.org)
California

"The services and programs revealed in the book are astounding. I only wish I knew about them earlier when I struggled as a caregiver to my mother—alone and with no support. I had no idea how much was available to me. This book is a MUST for any caregiver. Thank you Dr. Superson for the intensive research required to make this book possible. It will help so many."
Dr. Mary Meadows—Naturopath, Teacher, Author
Arizona

"Amazing resource guide that will no doubt save people time and money! All the research has been done with easy to access links right at your fingertips. Free products, services and programs are available to people if they only knew where to look. This guide is easy to use and can benefit Caregivers, Hospital Case Managers, Social Workers, Seniors, and Veterans."
Judy McTaggart—RN, BSN, CCM
Texas

"This Resource Guide saves so much time and energy when searching for needed information. It is well compiled, deeply thought out, and well organized. The programs, services, and products can easily save thousands of dollars every year—in addition to ways to be paid while caring for a family member. Not knowing what is available, what to ask for, or who to even talk to, can be overwhelming and stressful. Having this Resource Guide has been a blessing beyond words. If you don't already own a copy, you will wish you had! Thank you! Thank you! Thank you again!"
Juliana Olague—Experienced Caregiver
New Mexico

"Dr. Superson is a seasoned caregiver and professional who has taken the time to share the resources and 'secrets' she has discovered. No other book has everything you need in one convenient place including websites, contact information, and what specific services to ask for. This book is priceless!"
Diane Carbo—RN
Pennsylvania

"This Resource Guide is truly amazing and incredible. Dr. Superson has incorporated her practical— often humorous—time and money saving tips in a simple yet thorough guide. With easy, step-by-step instructions to obtain information FAST, any person can start saving money immediately. To say "I Love It" is an understatement! I know so many people who can benefit from this information. People have no idea how many vitally important programs, services, and products are available they may not be aware of, or even considered. We're talking about THOUSANDS OF DOLLARS here!
Jacque Zoccoli—Networking Coach, Collaboration Specialist
Arizona

"I have known Camille for over 25 years. We have compared notes over the years on caregiving, as we both cared for ailing parents. I only wish I had this book at that time, as it would have made life so much easier. Her book gives every important resource a caregiver will need. Not only are there resources for the one being cared for, but for the caregiver as well. I couldn't believe how many free or low-cost services are available. This book is an absolute MUST HAVE for anyone caring for an elderly parent, or a disabled child or adult. If only I knew then what I know now!"
Donna Czubernat
Illinois

"I have an aging parent who will need my help very soon. I had no idea what steps to take, who to call, or what to ask for. The thought of having to do any of this, was overwhelming. In my experience, it has always been the questions I did not know to ask, that lead to poor decisions and actions. Having all the information in one convenient place, with quick, easy, and simple-to- follow directions—makes this book a MUST for any caregiver. I was surprised to learn how many of the programs and services are free, making it so easy to protect your time, your money, your health, and your emotional wellbeing. I am grateful to own a copy!"
Craig Quaglia—MTPT, LMT
Illinois

"This Resource Guide helped me through to the last days of my father's life. It has truly been a blessing and was like having your best friend at your side all along the way. Dr. Camille has poured her heart into this lovely book, offering the vital information necessary to provide the vast array of resources that helped me transform caregiving into a compassionate, loving art form."
Sarah Moore
New Mexico

Essential Resource Guide
for Caregivers

Save Time...
Save Money...
Save Your Sanity!!!

Dr. Camille S. Superson

Double Infinity Publishing

Scottsdale, AZ

Essential Resource Guide for Caregivers
Save Time... Save Money... Save Your Sanity!!!

©2016, 2017 (2nd Edition), 2018 (3rd Edition), 2019 (4th Edition), 2020 (5th Edition), 2021 (6th Edition)
by Dr. Camille S. Superson

Double Infinity Publishing
Scottsdale, AZ 85252

ISBN: 978-0-578-85950-7 (paperback)

Also available in Kindle Digital

You may contact Dr. Superson by writing to her at the following address:
P.O. Box 2044
Scottsdale, AZ 85252

To book Dr. Superson as your next speaker and / or for bulk orders, you may contact her directly at Camille@DrCamilleSuperson.com, or call toll free **(844) 780-9962**.

DEDICATION

What a privilege to be raised by two people whose word was their honor;
where a handshake was better than a contract;
where being of service to others was an everyday occurrence;
where words weren't preached, but lived in deeds performed and as examples
to be emulated;
where every animal imaginable somehow found a home;
and with their passing, a huge void was felt by so many...

This book is dedicated to my parents, Helen and Mitchell Superson.

Their rich legacy also included a stroke and leukemia, and the challenges
faced in finding all the resources they needed during their respective illnesses.

Without them, this book would have never been written, and
Thousands of individuals, just like you, would not have benefited from many
*of the viable (and often **FREE**) products, services, and programs discovered both*
before and after their deaths.

They are the true heroes!

Their legacy of serving others continues indirectly—as the struggles faced,
and the lessons learned, transformed into a gift to help other caregivers
find many of the unknown, untapped, and difficult
to find resources contained in this book.

TABLE OF CONTENTS

PREFACE

I have played many roles in the course of my life. However, *nothing* compares to the vitally important role I was about to play when I became the full-time caregiver to both of my parents.

Like many of you, I was not at all prepared for my new role, and the adventure that was to unfold.

First, a little bit of history…

My parents were vibrant, high-energy contributors to society, whose minds were sharp and alert. They reached their early 70s and 80s with relatively good health, so becoming a 24-hour / 7-day-a-week caregiver to both was totally unexpected, and something I simply never considered.

My caregiver journey began when my mother suffered a severe stroke that left her bedbound, almost completely paralyzed, and totally reliant on others to get through the day.

Several years later, I learned my father had leukemia.

After my mother's stroke, I began to travel back and forth between Chicago and Michigan. Every weekend—Friday through Sunday—I would drive from *my* home to the home of my parents to help and assist in my mother's care. The traveling temporarily ceased when I brought my mother home to live with me in Chicago.

A year-and-a-half later, my father decided to bring my mother back to Michigan, where he could again be close to her. He didn't want to leave the familiarity of his own home to join us, so traveling between both states again resumed. Soon, he too, became ill and hospitalized.

Without hesitation, I returned to Michigan to care for my mother while my father recuperated. I believed I would eventually return to my own home, never thinking this particular trip would be a permanent one.

Overnight, I had become a 24 / 7 caregiver to both parents.

My father now required his own hospital bed, along with a vast array of medical treatments. One hospital bed on the first floor, and another on the second floor, made for an interesting situation. I would have loved to have been a fly on the wall, observing myself as I would run up and down the stairs every day, caring for both of them.

I had become very resourceful in terms of juggling everything I needed to do in a day.

My father seemed to be getting better, when suddenly his condition took a turn for the worse. From this point on, everything began happening at lightning speed. His death caught me totally by surprise, and grief engulfed me like an unwelcomed visitor. You would have thought I might have been emotionally prepared for this. I assure you, I was *not*—not in the least!

Caring for my mother allowed me to divert my grief in a positive way—as caring for her helped to refocus my attention on her, rather than focus elsewhere.

As I continued to care for her needs—and although she could not speak—her nonverbal hand communication gave me solace and joy knowing that she understood my words. Her ability to move her right hand in response to 'yes' and 'no' questions enabled us to communicate, and it always delighted me as to how much she understood.

When the time came when she also left us, a huge void filled my heart. Not only was I missing *both* parents—after 10 years of caregiving—I was totally exhausted.

It had been a learn-as-you-go experience in so many ways, and shortly thereafter, I began to reflect on all I had learned. I knew there were other caregivers out there—just like *you*—who were also experiencing the same trials and tribulations I had.

I also knew I compiled some very valuable **FREE** resources during my time as a caregiver, and much of that information was not discovered until seven years into my caregiving journey. Life would have been so much easier, and the wallet a whole lot fatter, had I known this information from the onset.

I remember spending countless hours hunting and searching and calling for information to help both my parents and me. I remember being frustrated when I received incorrect or limited information—and frustrated even more when a stranger offered important, cost-saving information which could have been suggested by any number of government agency personnel.

From personal experience, I know the roads you have yet to travel, and the challenges you may be facing every day. Having enough money to care for your loved one, and finding the time to search for the information you need and require, are often at the top of a caregiver's list, and only adds to the stress.

As I began writing and further researching and compiling this Resource Guide, I began discovering and uncovering even *more* additional information besides what I already knew—sometimes taking hours or days to uncover—including those resources often difficult to find.

I felt the need to simplify this material in order to make the information quick and easy for you to access, and with minimal effort. I wanted to direct you to *specific* areas on websites, so you didn't have to waste your time reading the volumes of information that didn't pertain to your immediate needs.

You now hold in your hands, the result of all my searching. It is a very special gift that will guide you to many valuable products, services, programs, information, and tips—all to help make your caregiving experience a more positive and uplifting one. Now that you know many of these resources are **FREE** to you, it will allow you to breathe a little easier, and provide hope and support during a time when you may need it most.

Remember, by not having to waste needless hours on the Internet searching for things, this Resource Guide will also help provide additional windows of time to be with those you love. The quality time you will be able to share with your loved one(s), might just become one of the greatest gifts they will ever receive from you!

Stay Blessed… Hang Tough… and Savor the Moments…

Know that I am here to support you and cheer you on!

Camille

P.S. As you read through the material, you will discover this Resource Guide is not only for caregivers. TIME and MONEY can be saved by EVERYone—in so many areas—on products and services you may already be using or needing every day!

Dr. Camille S. Superson

INTRODUCTION

Two of the most pressing concerns most caregiver families face, involve TIME and MONEY, and the pending disappearance of both. This becomes even more apparent as time goes by.

Did you know you may be squandering these two precious commodities without even knowing it?

What *if* you could change that?

What *if* you were able to keep more money in your wallet?

What *if* you were able to add more hours to your day?

The fact is you *can*... if you only knew how!

As you read on, the situations below may sound very familiar to you.

If you are like most caregivers, you may not be prepared for the journey that lies before you. Most people aren't. If you have been caring for a loved one for an extended period of time, I know you can easily relate.

Juggling family, a personal life, and a job you may have to quit while caring for your loved one, can easily take its toll. Quitting your job or cutting back on hours will only add to your financial hardship. Money always seems to be reallocated toward unexpected expenses or emergencies, and simple items that had no previous use, now have become staples in your life.

How about your *time*?

Do you often feel there is never enough time in the day to accomplish all you need to do?

Are you spending hours on the Internet searching for the help you need to care for your loved one?

By the end of the day, are you so exhausted, you wish a little genie would appear to help you out?

The good news is... your wish has been heard, and your genie is here! (That's me!) ☺

Imagine saving *thousands* of dollars and *hundreds* of hours of time—precious time that can never be replaced.

Imagine having everything you need conveniently at your fingertips.

Imagine having a lot more cash in your wallet when you discover how many products, services and programs may be available to you for **FREE**!

You no longer have to imagine, as this resource guide will become your close and valued friend. It will become a reference you will use time and time again. You will find yourself keeping it close by, and reaching for it more often than you ever thought you would.

Thousands of hours were devoted to researching, compiling, and organizing this information so you do not have to waste your valuable time searching for it yourself. Much of the information is difficult to find if you don't know where to look—and more importantly—if you aren't even aware this information is available to you in the first place. It doesn't matter if you are caring for an elderly parent, a veteran, or a child with disabilities or special needs. You will find valuable resources you can use immediately— even for yourself!

The websites, contact information, and the *specific* programs and services to look up or ask for are all provided for you. By using my easy-to-follow instructions, you will be able to bring up the local information you will need, right to your doorstep (no matter where you live in the United States). Contact information is also provided for products as well. These resources can easily save thousands of dollars every year, and you will stop squandering both your time and money away needlessly. You will see how quickly the dollars can add up, and you will be amazed how easy it is to do.

With that said, let's begin...

HOW TO USE THIS RESOURCE GUIDE

This Resource Guide is not written to be read from cover to cover like a novel. It is a book similar to an old fashioned 'Yellow Pages'—where you look up what you may want or need, obtain the contact information, then get the 'stuff.'

The 'stuff' is like finding the mother-load of a sunken treasure ship that had been buried in the ocean—minding its own business—until one day, a deep-sea diver decided to hunt for the treasures.

And treasures they are!

The golden nuggets of information found within these pages are priceless. I'm sure you could find many of them if you looked long enough, and hard enough. The fact is, most of you have no idea what many of these golden nuggets even are, let alone where to look to find them.

Hi, I'm Camille... your deep-sea diver at your service! (Who has a day job serving as 'personal genie' for caregivers with special wishes.) 😃

I hope that brought a little smile to your face, as a sense of humor is a good thing to have on those days when things may not be going as well as planned. A sense of humor will become one of the most important survival tools in your caregiving adventure.

Having been a caregiver for over a decade, I think I have *some* experience in the 'hunt and find it' scenario when it comes to this caregiving thing.

At the beginning of my personal tour of duty, I thought of myself as a fairly intelligent person. I was rudely awakened by how little I actually knew in this caregiver arena. Trying to find all the 'stuff' I needed between juggling all the daily caregiver responsibilities, stole hours of my life, and time away from those I loved most.

Sure, I was able to find *some* of the 'stuff'—only to be shocked and angered by the fact it was only the tip of the iceberg, and I had literally wasted thousands of dollars needlessly by not having more crucial information.

Having lived through the experience (barely), I came out with a mission. That mission was to help caring individuals like yourself steer clear of icebergs, and provide the resources you need *before* you even knew you needed them.

Do I know what I'm talking about? You bet! As the saying goes... *"Been there! Done that!"*...with full hands-on experience that was *not* for the weak of spirit, or faint of heart.

So, I guess I qualify as a true veteran in the field. I know what you will need to survive the experience without losing your health and sanity.

Look around. Check out fellow caregivers. Ask them how they're doing and most of them will tell you how stressed and overwhelmed they are with this new role… and many of them have only been at it for a few months!

Keeping this in mind, let's get back to how to use this Resource Guide.

My suggestion is to take this book with you whenever you can, so you can read it during any odd or spare moments during the day when you are not at home (like at lunchtime, on the train while you travel back and forth to work, or while you are waiting for an appointment).

Initially, thumb through the book relatively quickly to get a general feel as to what's inside. You may also want to have a small note pad or a few index cards to tuck in the book while away from home. Jot down ideas or reference pages, and refer to them later when you are able to relax and follow up more thoroughly.

There is no 'fluff' included, so take your time when you start investigating the topics most pressing to you. When you find a topic of interest, check that topic first. Read the section thoroughly, hop on your computer, then follow the links or make the phone calls.

While investigating these topics on the websites I provide, you will notice additional information on the site that may pique your interest and curiosity. Do not gloss over them, as you may wish to glean more information at a later date. Simply keep focused on the most pressing issues first—take a few notes regarding the websites of interest—and develop a simple filing system where you are able to retrieve and review the information later. You may also want to highlight or make notes directly in the Resource Guide.

Checklists are also provided at the end of each section for you to duplicate and write down information.

Websites are dynamic, and may change a bit from time to time. The 'keywords' or specific names for programs, often remain consistent enough to bring up the information you are looking for. What to look for on a particular website is clearly spelled out in this Resource Guide, and contain phone numbers and additional contact information, should you need them.

Again, remember to make additional copies of all the checklists at the back of each section, so you can document your findings.

I think you'll be as amazed as I was, as to what you will discover!

Your goal is to eventually read everything in this Resource Guide. It won't be hard to do, because it will be like opening your birthday presents, and getting even *more* than you asked for. You will begin to discover programs and services you may not even know exist, or even considered checking into—yet these resources may be fully available to you and your family. Many of them are **FREE**!

One of the biggest money robbers for me was discovering I overpaid over $13,000 for my mother's briefs / diapers & more, when I could have received them **FREE**! Then there was the overpayment of almost $6,000 for two funerals because I didn't know one simple strategy. Let's not forget the thousands of dollars I overpaid for prescriptions, doctor visits, home repairs, property taxes and more—simply because I didn't know there were multiple programs that could pay for them.

The wallet emptied, and the money disappeared like a thief in the night.

I would have given anything to have had a Resource Guide like this one when I was a caregiver.

Trust me! You Need To Know This Information!

Not because I wrote the book, but because you do not have the time or money to waste frivolously. In no time flat, you may receive many services you never considered, respite care you desperately need, and products you need and use every day… all for **FREE**! (If not completely **FREE**, then deeply discounted for sure!)

All the hard work is done for you. All you have to do is look things up in one convenient place, rather than spending hours on the Internet searching in a vacuum. You will learn what to ask for, how and where to make contact, and who to speak to.

How easy is that?

So get busy—*right now*—and start collecting some of the awesome treasures that are just waiting to be discovered!

Camille

P.S. This Resource Guide is not geared to any *specific* disease—as the resources included (products, services, and programs) are those *essential t*o everyone, with my prime focus on those resources that are **FREE**, or deeply discounted.

Also, learn how to actually get *paid* to care for a family member!

Most caregivers are not aware these options even exist or may even be available to them.

Now you know! ☺

GOVERNMENT AGENCY RESOURCES

*Note that websites (especially Government websites) are always dynamic and changing, and the information & programs may vary and change accordingly. Simply be aware of this fact when you make contact. Mention the program or service you are looking for, and the person you are speaking with should be able to guide and direct you.

Specific information on available resources and programs from government agencies is often difficult to find without secret passwords.

This section contains the secret passwords you will need.

😃

*"And when he came to the aforesaid rock
and to the tree whereon Ali Baba had hidden himself, and he had made sure
of the door, he cried in great joy, "Open, Sesame!" The portal yawned wide
at once and Kasim went within and saw the piles of jewels and treasures
lying ranged all around."*

—Ali Baba and the 40 Thieves

OBAMACARE
(also known as the Affordable Care Act)

Health insurance coverage under the ObamaCare / Affordable Care Act (ACA) plan is complex and constantly changing. These changes will continue to unfold until 2022, *unless new healthcare laws are implemented under our current administration.*

Under the current ACA program, all Americans are required to obtain health insurance. This insurance is generally obtained by direct purchase, through an employer, or through government programs such as Medicaid and Medicare (unless you qualify for exemption status and certain criteria are met).

Enrollment dates for 2021: October 15 to December 7, 2020. Effective February 15th, 2021, President Joe Biden directed the federally run HealthCare.gov to reopen enrollment from Feb. 15 through May 15 for certain states. Please check your state to see if it is reopened.

As of January 1, 2019 - the tax penalty has been eliminated, should you choose not to enroll.

If you sign up online from the **obamacarefacts.com** website, there is a link on the website called **"Health Insurance Marketplace"** to enroll.

Insurance companies may bid for your business at that site. You may be able to obtain a tax credit for a portion of the premiums purchased, if your income qualifies.

There are so many variables in this program, it is best to either call directly, or type in specific 'keywords' into the search area on the website (found at the top of the page).

For example: If you are looking for "exemptions," type the word **"exemptions"** into the search area, and you should receive answers to your questions.

obamacarefacts.com

healthcare.gov (for additional information)

(800) 508-6754

MEDICARE

Medicaid and Medicare: **cms.gov**

Medicare: **medicare.gov**

Qualifications:

- 65 years of age and eligible for Social Security
- Spouse of someone 65 years of age who is eligible for Medicaid and Social Security
- Have end-stage renal disease or other eligible disability, regardless of age

Note: Even if you do not plan on retiring by age 65, it is advisable to contact Social Security three months prior to your 65th birthday to enroll in Medicare.

Guidelines:

- To enroll without penalty, you must apply between the three months prior to the month of your 65th birthday and the three months after the month of your 65th birthday, totaling a seven month period
- If you do not apply by your enrollment deadline, but later decide to enroll in Medicare Part B (see Medicare Part B, below):
  - You will have to wait until the next open-enrollment period (January 1st – March 31st)
  - It will not be effective until the following July 1st
  - There is a 10% penalty for each 12-month period you could have enrolled in Medicare but did not
  - You will have to pay the penalty for as long as you are enrolled in Medicare Part B, and twice the number of years you could have had Part A, but did not sign up

If you have difficulty paying your Medicare premiums, you may qualify for assistance.

- When you are on the Medicare website, type **"How do I apply for Medicare Savings Programs?"** into the search area, to see if you qualify

Note:

- Medicare may / will undergo vast changes regarding what they will or will not cover in the future under the current healthcare law (known as Obamacare)

- Billions of dollars in anticipated cuts to the program have been debated in recent years

- For now, seniors are still able to obtain a variety of benefits through the Medicare program

Important Medicare Benefit:

At this time, everyone who is on Medicare qualifies for one FREE comprehensive wellness exam annually. This means that it is entirely FREE, with no deductibles, and no co-pays. Many people are not aware of this benefit, so be sure to take advantage of it while it is still available to you.

Is Medicare a little confusing and difficult to understand? There is a mini-webinar on the website **caregiveraction.org** *that provides one of the BEST explanations regarding all aspects of Medicare. It is presented in short, bite sized, easy to understand segments, with graphics & visuals to help explain each area. From the website select the* **Toolbox** *tab at top of page. It will bring you to the* **Family Caregiver Toolbox.** *Select the blue box that says,* **"Video Series-Understanding Medicare."** *This should help answer many of the questions you may have.*

Medicare Part A: (Hospital Insurance)

Premiums:

There is no 'per-month' premium, because you or your spouse paid Medicare taxes while working (this is most common, and often referred to as "premium-free Part A"). If you pay for Medicare Part A, you may pay up to $471 per month, depending on the total quarters of work history—with those working less than 30 quarters paying the maximum amount. Those working 40 or more quarters pay nothing. It is important to contact Social Security for more details.

Covers:

- *Inpatient Hospital Stay (up to 90 days)*

  You Pay:

  - $1,484 deductible per each benefit period

  - $0 for days 1- 60; $371 per day for days 61-90 of each benefit period

- $742 per day for "lifetime reserve days" for days 91-150 of each benefit period—with a maximum of 60 reserve days per lifetime
- Beyond these 60 lifetime reserve days, you pay all costs

- *Blood*
  - **FREE** in most cases if the hospital receives it **FREE** from a blood bank
  - If hospital must purchase, you pay for the first three units in a given calendar year

- *Skilled Nursing Home Care (up to 100 days)*
  - Must be in the hospital for at least three days to be able to move into a skilled nursing home facility
  - Always check for any other requirements, as Medicare is undergoing constant changes during the next decade

  You Pay:
  - $0 for first 20 days each benefit period
  - Up to $185.50 co-pay per day for days 21 – 100 of each benefit period
  - All cost beyond day 101for each benefit period
  - Coverage may be affected if there is any break in care, if you stop receiving skilled nursing care from the facility, or leave the skilled nursing facility altogether.
  - If your break in skilled care lasts more than 30 days, a new three-day hospital stay is needed to qualify for additional skilled care. If the break lasts more than 60 consecutive days, you are able to renew your benefits up to 100 days of skilled care coverage.

- *Home Healthcare*

  You Pay:
  - $0 for Home Healthcare services
  - 20% of the Medicare-approved amount for durable medical equipment

- *Hospice Care*

  You Pay:
  - $0

- Co-pay of up to $5 for outpatient prescription drugs for pain and symptom management only
- Up to 5% of the Medicare-approved amount for inpatient respite

Note: Medicare does cover Hospice Care in the home unless you need care in an inpatient facility… then the hospice team will make arrangements for your stay at an inpatient facility.

Medicare Part B: (Medical Insurance)

Premiums:

- Average premium $148.50 per month for 2021
  - May be automatically deducted from social security check (this amount is often lower for those already on Medicare, as their current net check can-not be less than what they are already receiving)
- The premium is higher if modified adjusted gross income (MAGI) is greater than $88,000 per individual, or $176,000 per couple
- New higher MAGI (added in 2019)—$500,000 per individual, or $750,000 per couple
- May be as high as $504.90 per month depending on income
- There is an annual $203 deductible, plus 20% of Medicare approved charges

Covers:

- *Medical expenses (up to 80%)*
- *Laboratory Fees*
- *Outpatient Hospital Treatment (up to 80%)*
- *Blood*
  - **FREE** if received from a blood bank, with an additional co-pay for processing on every unit given (which is different from Part A)

OR

- You pay for first three units in a calendar year if provider must purchase for you—co-pay for processing also applies, and amount paid is applied toward deductible (a bit different from Medicare Part A)

- *Durable Medical Equipment (up to 80% Medicare approved amount)*

- *Diabetic Supplies (including test strips, monitors, insulin and more)*

- *Preventive Health Services and Screenings—many are **FREE**, depending on service*

- *Physician Office Visits (up to 80% Medicare approved amount)*

- *Physician Charges (up to 80% Medicare approved amount)*

- *Physical Therapy & Speech-Language Pathology Services combined (80% of $2,110 before requiring medical necessity to continue treatment, and no dollar limit if treatment deemed medically necessary)*

- *Occupational Therapy (80% of $2,110 before requiring medical necessity to continue treatment, and no dollar limit if treatment deemed medically necessary)*

Social Security and the Centers for Medicare & Medicaid Services have worked together to create special state programs to help pay Medicare Part B premiums and other medical costs. Call to see if you qualify for assistance.

Medicare Part C (also known as the Medicare Advantage Plan)

Medicare Part C will no longer be available after January 1, 2020 to newly eligible individuals. Those eligible for Medicare Part A prior to 2020 will continue to have this option available.

- Obtained through private insurance

- Covers everything original Medicare covers

- Combination of Medicare Part A, B, and D (prescription coverage)

- Covers additional benefits original Medicare does not cover

- Not all plans cover same extra benefits—so read descriptions before deciding on a company

- Advantage plans are either Preferred Provider Organizations (PPOs) or Health Maintenance Organizations (HMOs)

Durable Medical Equipment

Effective January 2019, some Medicare Advantage plans may reimburse part or all of the costs for home modifications to assist or aid the elderly to keep them safe. These home modifications can play a vitally important role in preventing accidents and falls by enhancing stability and balance, and ease of mobility throughout the home.

Medicare Part B has always paid a large portion of the medical equipment charges for wheelchairs, walkers, hospital beds, and several other durable medical equipment necessities—yet most home modifications were not covered at all by straight Medicare.

Those of you who have certain Medicare Advantage plans can now be totally or partially reimbursed for the following items. Contact your insurance company to check.

Some important items that have been added are:

- Wheelchair ramps

- Widening of door frames and entrances to accommodate wheelchairs

- Handrails / guard rails

- Kitchen modifications to adjust countertop heights and more…

- Bathroom safety modifications including:

  - Grab bars

  - Walk in showers

  - Modifications to keep a person safe

> Contact information for Medicare:
>
> **(800) 633-4227**
>
> **(877) 486-2048 TTY users**

Medicare Part D

This program provides limited prescription coverage through private insurance companies. For those who choose to enroll, there may be a monthly premium.

- Medicare Part D was initially set up for individuals with NO prescription coverage

- If you have your own private insurance, it is often better than what you will receive from Medicare Part D

- If you have your own private insurance, you do not have to enroll in Medicare Part D

- If you do enroll in Medicare Part D and have Medicare Advantage insurance (Medicare Part C), you could lose your private insurance

- Often difficult to requalify for private insurance—you *will* lose it after enrolling in Medicare Part D, are retired, and if received through a former employer or union

- Maximum deductible for stand-alone Part D prescription drug plans is $445 for 2021

- "Donut hole" closed in 2020

  - Pay only 25% of all brand name and generic drug costs (versus 100% in the past) – until catastrophic threshold ends

- Out-of-pocket threshold increased from $6,350 to $6,550 in 2021

Opting for Medicare Part D

It is VERY important that you enroll with the policy that fits your individual and specific prescription needs.

- Consult with your insurance agent first, especially if your medication is generic

- Check with your local pharmacies for the best prices on generics

  - Many pharmacies give a 30-day supply for $4 or a 90-day supply for $10 (or something very similar), so check there first

    o There are several hundred generic drugs that may be available on this program

    Pharmacies that participate in this program are listed below. Please check with your local pharmacies to see if they participate in this program. Not all pharmacies cover the same generics—make sure you price-check several.

    - Walmart

    - Sam's Club

    - Costco

    - Winn-Dixie

    - Walgreens

    - Check other pharmacies as well...

    - There *may* be an annual fee, depending on the pharmacy

- When meeting with an insurance agent representing Medicare Part D, be sure to present a list of all medications you are taking

  - Include the name, strength, and monthly quantity

  - Include the monthly cost you are currently paying for each prescription

  - Be sure you check to see if any of your generic medications are listed on any of the $4 / $10 programs listed previously

- You can always sign up for Medicare Part D in the future, should your medications change—just know there *will* be a penalty imposed under the current law

- You *may* be charged a penalty down the road for every month you were eligible for Medicare Part D and did not receive it (one percent of the national average of premiums per month, for every month not received—for the duration of your coverage)

Note: *Please check the **PRESCRIPTIONS** section of this Resource Guide (**page 143**). In that section, there are ways to obtain **FREE** or **discounted** medications by using a multitude of Discount Prescription Cards or various prescription programs that provide **FREE** medications.*

*Discount Prescription Cards may often be used in conjunction with other insurance prescription plans for even further **discounts**.*

If you do *not* have the resources to pay for your prescriptions, Medicare also offers other alternatives based on need.

- For those who qualify, there is a monthly cap of $3.70 for generics and $9.20 for brand name medications

- You must be enrolled in Medicare Part D to partake in this program

- Please call the Medicare or Social Security numbers below to see if you qualify.

The program is called:
"Limited Income Subsidy" (LIS) or "Extra Help"

(800) 633-4227 Medicare direct number

(800) 772-1213 Social Security direct number

Medicare Part F

Beginning January 1, 2020, Medigap plans (Plan F or high deductible version Plan F) sold to newly eligible individuals will no longer cover the Medicare Part B deductible.

If you are already enrolled in either Medicare Part C or Medicare Part F prior to January 1, 2020, you may keep your plan(s).

Finding the Best Drug Plan for You

Medicare: **medicare.gov**

If you have any difficulty finding what you need, you can always contact Medicare directly at:

(800) MEDICARE – (800-633-4227)

Medicare will undergo vast changes over the next decade as long as the current healthcare law remains in effect. These changes may include the Medicare website, and you may need to call Medicare directly for specific questions on the availability of various programs.

If you are looking for Medicare programs to help pay for your prescriptions, type in any of the following phrases in the search box on the **medicare.gov** website:

"Prescription Drug Coverage"

"Medicare Prescription Drug Finder"

"Learn More About the Plans in Your Area"

This should bring up various links for you to check for more detailed information, including how to proceed further. Simply follow directions on the various sites, or call Medicare directly for further assistance.

By viewing and comparing the various programs, you can choose the best plan for you. One of the most discouraging factors for many individuals who enrolled in Medicare Part D was the **"donut hole."**

*The donut hole was eliminated from ALL current plans in 2020
for both generic and brand name drugs.
There may be additional changes which can affect drug costs in the
coming years—so watch for them.*

Hopefully, any changes will be good ones.

Note: *ALWAYS compare the 'cash' cost of your generic medication at various pharmacies that offer the $4 / $10 programs (or something similar) for 30- and 90-day supplies. Many of your medications may be on that list. Even when you sign up for Medicare Part D, you will still be able to pay the cash price for medications that may be on the 30 / 90-day generic list IF the medication(s) are not covered on your plan, or if the cash price for these generics are less than the co-pay amounts for the same generic(s) on your plan.*

STATE Health Insurance Assistance Program (SHIP)

- State program obtains funding from the federal government to provide **FREE** one-on-one local health coverage counseling and assistance to people with Medicare and their families

- Some states call their SHIP program by another name

- To find your state's SHIP program:
    - From the website **SeniorsResourceGuide.com**
        - Scroll down page to find your state website and hotline number

- If you are eligible for Medicare—you are eligible for SHIP

MEDICAID

Medicaid and Medicare: **cms.gov**

Medicaid is a government health insurance program for **low-income** families. There are eligibility requirements of minimal income and assets. Check with your local state agency for specific qualifications.

Medicaid: **medicaid.gov**

- From the website, type **"Contact information for Medicaid"** into the search area at the top and select **Search**
    - Select the first link on the page displayed (**Contact Us-Medicaid.gov**)
    - To the right of the page find **"Contact Your State Medicaid Agency"** where there will be a dropdown menu to find your state
    - **Select your state** and hit **Go**
        - A list of contact information to various programs, questions, and a variety of other information will become available regarding your state
        - Every state varies as to what information is provided on the site
        - You should be able to obtain a phone number (or phone numbers) to contact someone to help you with your questions and qualifications

        At times, it may be challenging to find a phone number, so do not be surprised if that's the case when you are attempting to contact a particular state. Frustrating, I know...

Covered expenses included:

- Physician visits
- Laboratory tests
- Hospital stays
- Diagnostic tests
- Nursing home care
- Money
- Prescription coverage
- Children's health insurance
- Food stamps
- And more...

AREA AGENCIES ON AGING

The National Area Agencies on Aging (AAA) provides many valuable resources and benefits for the elderly so they are able stay in their homes.

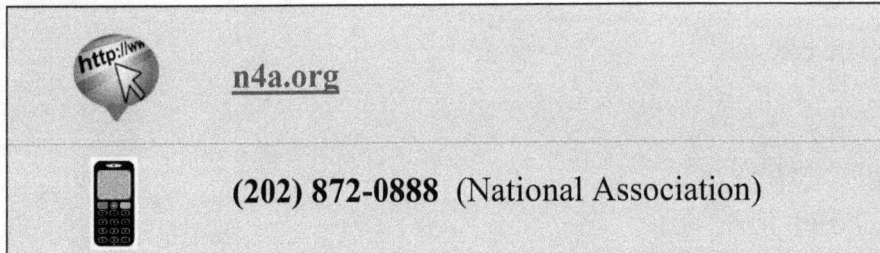

n4a.org

(202) 872-0888 (National Association)

To receive the program benefits listed on the website, you must contact your **LOCAL** Area Agency on Aging. This information can be found by simply entering **your city and state** OR **zip code** in the area provided on the above website.

- Provides contact information and phone numbers for the organizations in the immediate area where you live

Each individual state has designed their own Area Agency on Aging (AAA) to address the needs of the elderly at the *local* level. These AAAs may be public or private nonprofit agencies.

The Purpose of AAA:

- Offers a multitude of services to help older Americans stay in their homes
- Many of these services are **FREE**
- Helps coordinate the services offered, and much more...

CAREFULLY READ THE INFORMATION BELOW

Area Agency on Aging (AAA) is a **generic** term, so the specific name for each *local* AAA will vary.

For example: The Southeast Michigan AAA is called "Area Agency on Aging 1-B" (AAA1-B), while another for Taylor Michigan is called "The Senior Alliance-1C." The name variations may not follow any particular pattern, so be aware these differences *do* exist.

These name variations may make it a little difficult to find the programs you are seeking. ***Check all the resources*** that come up when you enter your zip code from the website. This will provide more information should you need to call the agency with questions.

The AAA programs have specific requirements to qualify. Take the time learn what is offered from the local websites. **Call the numbers** provided to gather even more detailed information, then **document** everything on the checklist provided at the end of this section.

The examples provided on the next several pages, will show a cross section of possibilities to ask for. **Each state and each city may vary in what they provide, yet are often very similar**.

You may be pleasantly surprised with what you discover, as you perhaps had no idea as to how much is available to you. **Keep asking questions** when you call for more information. Remember to use the checklists provided to document your discoveries.

Eldercare Locator: <u>eldercare.acl.gov</u>

(800) 677-1116

More information about AAA may be available from the website above.

1. From the homepage, **enter your zip code** or **city and state** in the box provided.
2. Contact information for AAAs in your area, as well as other local services and programs will be provided.
3. See **Telephone Techniques** at the end of this section for guidelines to follow when making calls to the different agencies.
4. For a long list of valuable resources and categories that are *Topic Specific*, click the **Resources** tab at the top of the page. From that page, select the link from the left side of the page (under **Resources)** called **Helpful Links**.
5. Then select either **Federal Websites** or **Additional Links** for many valuable resources that provide these *Topic-Specific* services.
6. The **Federal Websites** link provides websites to many Federal programs and services.
7. The **Additional Links** link provides helpful non-profit websites that focus on eldercare and other important issues of concern. Select any of the following three (3) links for more information: **Aging Organizations, Health and Disease Specific Organizations,** or **End of Life.**

See the **Southeast Michigan Area Examples** on the following pages for an overview of the types of programs that *may* be available in your area.

Getting Started:

1. Contact your *local* AAA by telephone (see **page 27** for how to locate).

2. The agency will provide specific information regarding qualification requirements and support services for your *local* AAA.

3. *There may be additional information available and not shown on the website. Ask the person you are speaking with to send you written information on the available programs.*

The following pages show several examples of the services and programs offered in Southeast Michigan, and are not inclusive. Often programs can be moved, eliminated, or incorporated within other programs—as the parameters may change from time to time. The eligibility or services within a particular program may also change. These examples are provided as a guide ONLY, and know that some of the programs may now be incorporated within other programs, or may be a stand-alone provided service.

The person you will speak to from AAA 1-B will often be able to give immediate answers to your questions when you provide any of the key words listed in the example programs.

This information is included for use as a reference only, so you can see the types of programs being offered. Programs in your area may vary slightly—however, many may be similar.

While this is likely NOT your local area, the examples provided on the following pages are presented as a guide to help you when you call YOUR local contact number for more information regarding similar programs. THESE ARE EXAMPLES ONLY.

SOUTHEAST MICHIGAN AAA EXAMPLES

AAA 1-B

The agency providing services to many areas in southeast Michigan is the "Area Agency on Aging 1-B (AAA 1-B)." It is a nonprofit organization.

AAA 1-B provides points of access to care for individuals who are 60 years of age and older, their caregivers, and adults with disabilities living in Livingston, Macomb, Monroe, Oakland, St. Clair Shores, and Washtenaw counties in the state of Michigan.

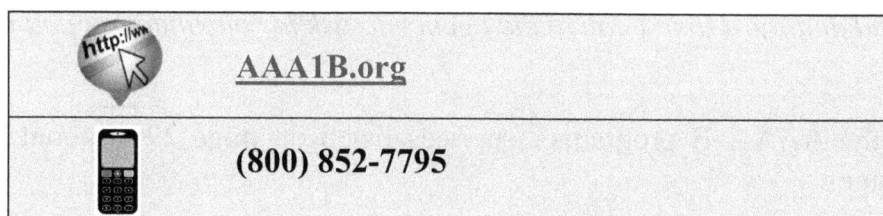

http://w **AAA1B.org**	
📱	**(800) 852-7795**

You will want to find the website for YOUR local area (see **page 27**). In addition to the programs or services listed on the following pages, there are more contact numbers and programs listed on the AAA1-B website.

While every area of the country offers various programs, they are often very similar. Check the information for services offered in *your* local AAA.

Possible Programs / Services Available from AAA1-B

1. MI Choice Medicaid Waiver Program
2. Community Living Program
3. Medicare / Medicaid Assistance Program
4. In-Home Services Programs
5. Out-of-Home Respite Referral Service
6. Rapid Response Respite (Respite care for 'burnt out' caregiver situations)
7. Nursing Facility Transition Services
8. Information and Assistance

SOUTHEAST MICHIGAN AAA EXAMPLES (continued)

When calling YOUR LOCAL AGENCY:

- *Ask for information about any and all programs available in your area*

- *Ask if they have any or all of the programs listed on the previous page, or something very similar*

- *Ask that written information to be sent to you*

- *Be persistent and continue to ask, as I received more program information the second and third time I called the agency to ask for clarification and updates*

Details for the AAA 1-B programs / services listed on **page 29** are contained on the following pages.

1. MI Choice Medicaid Waiver Program

The MI Choice Medicaid Waiver Program provides Medicaid covered services to qualified individuals 18+ requiring nursing home level of care.

This program is **NOT the regular Medicaid program**. While the individual may not qualify under regular Medicaid (financially), he / she may qualify for the **MI Choice Medicaid Waiver Program**.

Eligibility:

- Waitlist approximately 6 to 12 months… maybe less

- Age 18+ who qualifies for nursing home admission & financial guidelines met

- Nursing home resident who would be able to return home if supportive services were available & financial guidelines met

- Monthly income of $2,313 or less as an individual

- Individual assets do not exceed $2,000

- Assets exclude: owner occupied homes, primary vehicles, burial plots, and irrevocable funeral trusts

SOUTHEAST MICHIGAN AAA EXAMPLES (continued)

Program Services for Waiver:

- Homemaker services
- Respite care (in-home and out-of-home)
- Adult day care
- Transportation
- Medical equipment and supplies
- Chore Program services
- Personal emergency response systems
- Non-emergency medical
- MI Choice nursing services
- Private duty nursing
- Counseling
- Home-delivered meals (Meals on Wheels)
- Client / caregiver training
- Personal care and more…

Qualifying Steps:

- Telephone interview
- In-home assessment

SOUTHEAST MICHIGAN AAA EXAMPLES (continued)

Personal note from Camille about the "Waiver Program:"

When I obtained this resource, I found it to be invaluable! I discovered this program seven YEARS after my mother initially suffered her stroke—as no one from the agency, visiting nurses, or social workers ever informed me that this program was even available. Had it not been for a dear friend who was relentless in her inquiries, I may have never discovered it.

Some of the main benefits received from this program were:

- *Adult briefs / blue under pads, etc.—covered 100% as opposed to approximately $165 per month out-of-pocket. (That is a staggering figure of over $13,000 over seven years!)*

- *$1 medications versus her PPO co-pay of $4 to $20 per prescription*

- *Respite care provided to me on a limited basis every week*

At some point, after receiving updated information on the "Waiver Program," I asked to be transferred to another department so I could obtain updated information on the "Chore Program." The person giving information about the "Chore Program" was totally unaware the "Waiver Program" even existed.

*To add to the confusion, Michigan had both a "Chore Program" and a "Home Chore Program." The services provided were very different. One supplied outdoor services, like grass cutting and snow removal. The other provided a **FREE** hot water tank every few years, plus a line of credit for home maintenance. While caring for my parents—and having been on the program for several months—the hot water heater gave out, and it was nice to have it replaced for **FREE**!*

Your community may also have similar programs available, so always check.

*Because there are so many programs available, it is unlikely that one person will know all the different programs offered through **your** local Area Agency on Aging. You may run into the same difficulties I experienced. That is why you **must** be persistent! This Reference Guide will guide you through the steps, so you know in advance what information to inquire about. There are multiple options available here. Check for all that may be pertinent to you or your loved one.*

2. Community Living Program

Assists older adults with a variety of services to help them remain in their homes. These individuals pay a reduced rate for any care services they qualify for.

Eligibility:

- Age 60+ and needing in-home services

- Low income… payment is based on income

- Waitlist based on need or other criteria (you will need to ask for more information)

Program Services:

- Personal care

- Homemaking

- Respite for caregivers up to 10 hours per week

- Life Alert Alarm System

- Transportation and more…

Qualifying Steps:

- Telephone interview

- In-home assessment

3. Medicare / Medicaid Assistance Program

(800) 803-7174

Provides information and counseling on Medicare and Medicaid issues. There is no charge for this program.

SOUTHEAST MICHIGAN AAA EXAMPLES (continued)

Assistance includes information regarding:

- Medicare supplement insurance
- Long-term care insurance options
- Medicare prescription drug benefit programs
- Medicare Advantage Plans & more…

4. In-Home Service Programs

Provides home care assistance to older adults age 60+ who qualify through the Community Living Program, or those 18+ who qualify through the MI Choice Medicaid Waiver Program. Other options may also be available, so always ask what those options might be when speaking to someone from AAA 1-B.

Eligibility:

- Depends on the program the individual qualifies for (see above)
- Difficulty performing personal care / in-home tasks

Call AAA 1-B for more information:

(800) 852-7795

Program Services:

- Personal care
- Homemaker services
- Respite for caregiver & more…

Qualifying Steps:

- Telephone interview
- In-home assessment

5. Out-of-Home Respite Referral Service

Provides **respite for the caregiver**. Caregivers can make advanced reservations for care of their loved one through an Assisted Living Facility, an Adult Foster Care Facility, or Nursing Home. This service is in addition to Adult Day Care, and is listed here as a possible service to consider when there is a need to take an extended break to rest, recuperate, or simply take some time off to tend to your own personal needs or health concerns. Although this service is a private pay option in various parts of Michigan, some states offer this service on a sliding scale. It is important to check your individual state to see if this service is offered, and what the cost may be.

Eligibility:

- This is a private pay option and prices vary depending on the facility

- AAA 1-B will provide a list of facilities from their data base to help you find the right facility for your loved one

- Advanced notice must generally be given to the facility chosen

- Must check with the facility to make sure there is an open bed available

> Reservations / Eligibility Questions:
> Call AAA 1-B: **(800) 852-7795**

6. Rapid Response Respite Program

The primary focus of this program is to provide **immediate respite relief** to an **extremely burnt out caregiver**, no matter how old the caregiver may be. The care recipient must be age 60 and under.

SOUTHEAST MICHIGAN AAA EXAMPLES (continued)

Rapid Response Respite:

- Care recipient must be age 60 and under

- Primarily helps the caregiver experiencing caregiver burnout

- Provides up to 10 hours respite care per week

- Cost generally based on sliding scale

This program does *not* include the spouse or minor child. The AAA 1-B representative will be happy to speak with you and provide more details to see if you qualify for this service. Generally, there is NO WAITING LIST for those who qualify.

> Call AAA 1-B: **(800) 852-7795** for more information and an in-home assessment

7. Nursing Facility Transition Services

This program helps nursing home residents transition back into their home.

Eligibility:

- Nursing home residents age 18+

- Monthly income not greater than $2,199

- Assets no greater than $2,000

> Call AAA 1-B: **(800) 852-7795** for more information and an in-home assessment

SOUTHEAST MICHIGAN AAA EXAMPLES (continued)

Program Services:

- Assistance moving back into the community
- *May* provide one-time expense to acquire housing
- *May* provide utility hookup and deposits (cable not included)
- *May* provide one-time cleaning
- *May* provide one-time purchase of necessary items to set up household

> Call AAA 1-B: **(800) 852-7795** for a telephone interview to determine eligibility and what may or may not be covered

8. Information and Assistance

AAA 1-B helps locate services in southeast Michigan for older adults, disabled persons, and caregivers. It is designed to be a source for information to reduce confusion and increase support. There are thousands of service providers who provide a vast array of services throughout Southeast Michigan.

Information Provided:

- Personal care
- Prescription assistance
- Homemaker services
- Home-delivered meals
- Assisted living
- Care management
- And more...

- Senior center
- Home health agencies
- Adult day services
- Chore services
- Support groups
- Legal assistance

Remember, the previous examples are for Southeast Michigan Area Agency on Aging 1-B (AAA1-B)—which assist those living in Livingston, Macomb, Monroe, Oakland, St. Clair, and Washtenaw counties ONLY. Please follow the steps at the beginning of this Section (**page 26**), to find support telephone numbers for your *local* Area Agency on Aging.

FINANCIAL HELP FOR CAREGIVERS

The following websites have information on **caregiver benefits**. **Family caregivers** may be eligible for Medicaid, medications, food stamps, or other programs. Since many full-time caregivers sacrifice their careers to care for their loved ones—**there is a good possibility that you, as a family caregiver, may qualify for many of the programs available.**

CASH & COUNSELING programs allow family members to become paid caregivers to their loved ones. The programs are often called different names in different states.

Cash & Counseling

Cash & Counseling (C&C) helps people (generally disabled individuals and the elderly) direct and manage their own services, according to their individual needs. **C&C also provides cash allowances to family caregivers in most states. Please check your state for details.**

As of June 2015, there are now **four** different (C&C) / Consumer Directed care programs available. Forty-nine states have at least one or more of the following programs available:

- **Traditional Medicaid Waiver** (most common)

    - Recipients may choose their own home care agencies to obtain a caregiver

    - Family members (like the adult children of aging parents), or friends—can act as a 'home care agency,' and provide care services and personal assistance to the recipient

- **Non-Medicaid programs**

- **Veterans program / Veterans Directed Home and Community Based Services (VD-HCBS)**

    - Allows Veterans to choose their own caregivers (including family members) in place of those provided by the Veterans Administration (VA)

    - *Cannot* participate in both Medicaid C&C and VD-HCBS programs at the same time

    - War-time veterans *can* participate in the VD-HCBS program and still be eligible for the **Aid and Attendance** pension benefit [please refer to the **VETERAN & MILITARY** section of this guide (**page 180**) for more details on the **Aid and Attendance** pension benefit]

        o There *may* be a waitlist

        o You may choose another alternative VA Medical Center that does *not* have a waiting list

- This program is a joint effort of the VA and local Area Agencies on Aging (AAA)
  - You can contact either the VA or your local AAA to see if there is a program available in your area [please refer to **VETERAN & MILITARY section (page 176)** and your **local Area Agency on Aging (page 26)** of this Resource Guide for contact information]
  - Not available in every state (yet)—goal is to become available nationwide
- **Programs for Life Insurance Policy Holders**
  - **Life insurance policyholders who do not qualify for Medicaid,** can still use their life insurance policy to pay family members for caregiving
  - There are pros and cons with this option (see website link on **page 41**)
    - Pros and cons are explained in detail in the **Programs for Life Insurance Policy Holders** section of the website

All of the above Cash & Counseling programs allow family members (or friends, in some states) to become paid caregivers to their loved one(s).

Under the original C&C program, state monthly caps ranged from $500 to $4,000. These monthly allowances have now become much more diverse and broader, due to the addition of the new programs being offered. Maximum limits are yet to be determined. Amounts are generally determined by the amount of care the recipient requires. This amount may increase or decrease, depending on the needs of the recipient.

Note: Cash & Counseling programs are often called different names in different states—the most common (though not limited to) being "Consumer-Directed," "Participant-Directed," or "Self-Directed," program(s). Be persistent, and know the names may also change.

Examples:

THROUGH MEDICAID WAIVER: Most states have their own names for their Cash & Counseling Programs associated with a specific Medicaid waiver. In Washington it is called "New Freedom Program;" in Ohio, "PASSPORT;" in Montana, "Big Sky."

As you can see, the names of the programs may vary quite dramatically, depending on the state. This also applies to the names of the Non-Medicaid & Veterans Programs (VD-HCBS) as well.

Note from Camille:

It is important to actually CALL the contact number(s) provided for your state, and ask for the name of the Cash & Counseling program(s) in that state. Many of the people you will speak to may not know what the alternate name(s) are called. I called several states, and found this to be true before I finally received all the answers I needed. Each state also varies as to what qualifications are necessary for a family member (or friend) to actually receive the cash stipend. The link below should make it a little easier for you to find the actual name(s) of the C&C program(s) in your state. Then go to the very bottom of that page; find the program(s) available in your state; view the details of the programs; and call the number(s) provided.

Example: *In Illinois, the "Cash & Counseling" program is called "Community Care" program. It is part of the Illinois State Department on Aging (different from Area Agencies on Aging), and family members (or friends) may receive money to care for a loved one by meeting certain criteria. Criteria include having the recipient assessed for in-home care; family member (or friend) must obtain formal caregiver training; family member (or friend) must be hired by an outside caregiver agency; then the family member (or friend) is hired by recipient or recipient's family from the outside caregiver agency.* The **link below** will provide very detailed and specific information on every possible question you may have regarding C&C.

Type in **"Cash & Counseling Programs: Get Paid as a Family Caregiver"** into the address bar of your browser. The link should come up in the list of choices.

Then select the link:

"Cash & Counseling Programs: Get Paid as a Family Caregiver"

https://www.payingforseniorcare.com/paid-caregiver/cash-and-counseling-program

- Once you are on the website, scroll down (way down) to the very bottom of the page.

- Under the **List of Programs** area, you will find a list for the *Veterans, Insurance, Medicaid, and Non-Medicaid* C&C programs to obtain more information.

- For *Medicaid* and *Non-Medicaid* programs, **select your individual state** and the actual name of the program will appear at the top of the page with eligibility and descriptions provided for each program.

   Nursing home residents are NOT allowed to participate in this program.

   Some C&C programs allow assisted living residents to participate.

   Spouses are able to obtain cash for caring for a spouse in some states.
   Only a few states participate at this time.
   Check with your state to see if this program is offered.

Under the **"Family and Medical Leave Act"** (FMLA), a family caregiver is also entitled to up to 12 weeks of **unpaid leave** in a 12-month period without risk of job loss. You may also keep your employer-provided health insurance without termination of policy.

Keep your eye out for the **"Family and Medical Insurance Leave" (FAMILY)**, also referred to as the **"Paid Family Leave Act."** As of this writing, the bill has not passed, and is *NOT a federal law (yet)*. If passed, it **will provide up to 12 weeks of** *partial paid* **family leave** funded by employers and employee payroll contributions. ***Please refer to the LEGISLATION section of this Resource Guide for more information about the law.***

Please note: Your job is *not* guaranteed, as with the FMLA law of 1993. However, they are finding it benefits both employer and employee where these laws are currently in effect.

The following states are currently independently participating:

- **California**: 55% of income; up to $1075 / week; up to six weeks.

- **New Jersey**: 2/3 of weekly wage; up to $524 / week; up to six weeks.

- **Rhode Island**: 60% of weekly wage; up to $752 / week; up to four weeks.

- **Washington, D.C.**: Up to 90% of wages up to 1.5 x minimum wage—50% above that; up to $1000/week; up to eight weeks for new parents; up to six weeks for other family caregiving.

- **New York** was included, beginning:

  - **Phase I** January 1, 2018.

  - **Phase II** January 1, 2019: Up to 10 weeks **PAID** benefits in a 52-week period at 55% of average weekly rate.

  - **Phase III** January 1, 2020: Up to 10 weeks **PAID** benefits in a 52-week period at 60% of average weekly rate.

  - **Phase IV** January 1, 2021: 12 weeks **PAID** benefits in a 52-week period at 67% of average weekly rate.

- **Massachusetts:**

  - Most benefits begin January 2021.

  - Up to 20 weeks of job protected **PAID** leave for covered worker's own serious health condition.

  - **PAID** leave to care for a family member July 1, 2021.

    o Up to 12 weeks off per year.

  - Up to 26 weeks combined Medical / Family leave.

  - Maximum weekly benefit amount—$850 per week.

Medicare Programs

The Medicare website offers links to several programs that **may provide financial help**.

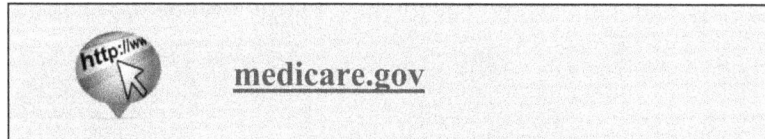

medicare.gov

Medicare Savings Programs (MSPs)

> If you have any difficulty finding what you need, you can always contact Medicare directly at:
>
> **(800) MEDICARE (800-633-4227)**
>
> Ask for the "Medicare Savings Programs."

Also remember that websites like Medicare are constantly changing. If so, type **"Medicare Savings Programs"** into the search area on the **Medicare.gov** website. It should bring up the information for you.

This program helps save money by paying deductibles, co-pays, some or all of your Medicare premiums, drugs, and more.

Apply for Extra Help

> If you have any difficulty finding what you need, you can always contact Medicare directly at:
>
> **(800) MEDICARE (800-633-4227)**
>
> Ask for the "Apply for Extra Help Program."

Also remember that websites like Medicare are constantly changing. If so, type **"Apply for Extra Help with Medicare Prescription Plan Costs"** in the search area on the **Medicare.gov** website. It should bring up the information for you.

This program offers help for prescription drugs to Medicare recipients who have a limited income and resources.

- This program is available through Social Security

- The amount you pay may vary from year to year, so always check for details

> **SocialSecurity.gov**
> OR
> **ssa.gov**
>
> **(800) 772-1213**
> 7 a.m. – 7 p.m. (Monday – Friday)
>
> **(800) 325-0778** TTY (toll free)

- Type **"APPLY for Extra Help with Medicare Prescription Plan Costs"** into the search area on the **SocialSecurity.gov** website and can apply online for this program

Pharmaceutical Assistance Program

If you have any difficulty finding what you need, you can always contact Medicare directly at: 1-800-MEDICARE (1-800-633-4227) and ask for the "Pharmaceutical Assistance Program."

Also remember websites like Medicare are constantly changing. If so, type **"Pharmaceutical Assistance Program"** in the search area on the **Medicare.gov** website. It should bring up the information for you.

This program is offered by drug manufactures to help those enrolled in Medicare Part D who are unable to pay for their medications, or experiencing financial hardship.

> **www.medicare.gov/pharmaceutical-assistance-program**

- An alphabetical index will appear

- Select the **first letter** of the drug you are looking for

- A menu of drug names will come up

- If you find your medication, select the **Details** link next to the drug name

- Pharmaceutical company information will then appear, including:

  - Drug program

  - Eligibility criteria

  - Benefits / Assistance

  - Website / contact information

  - **FREE** to those who qualify

STATE Pharmaceutical Assistance Program

This program helps pay drug plan premiums and / or other drug costs.

www.medicare.gov/pharmaceutical-assistance-program/state-programs.aspx

- Using the **Select a State** box—scroll to see if your state is eligible

- This program only offered in 21 states

- **Select your state** if it is on the list

- State information includes:

  - Program name

  - Telephone number

  - Who is eligible

  - Where to apply

  - Link to state website

  - Important notes

Explore National and Local Charitable Programs

Benefits Check Up is listed as the resource link. It identifies eligibility for several programs.

benefitscheckup.org

(800) 794-6559

9 a.m. – 5 p.m. EST (Monday – Friday)

- Type in your **zip code** and select the **Get Started** button once you are on the website

- Answer all the questions

- You may very easily quality for help and assistance to a vast array of products and services you may not be aware of, are entitled to, or simply do not know how to apply

- You will receive a report of programs you qualify for, which makes it easy for you to view at a glance

- Apply for these programs online, or submit an application form that can be printed out from your computer

- Benefits Checkup is a **FREE** service of the National Council on Aging (NCOA), especially those aged 55 and older

- There are over 2,000 programs and services available which are privately and government funded—saving thousands of dollars in everyday expenses

- Some expenses you may need help with include:

  - Utilities

  - Prescriptions

  - Meals / Food

  - Healthcare

  - Housing

  - Legal services

  - Taxes

  - In-Home Services

  - More…

Government Benefits

Benefits.gov is designed to provide improved and personalized Internet access to government benefits and assistance programs quickly and easily.

The website is exceptionally easy to navigate.

This is a website for everyone to check out, no matter what your background or current situation. There are many opportunities here you may not be aware of, yet may qualify for.

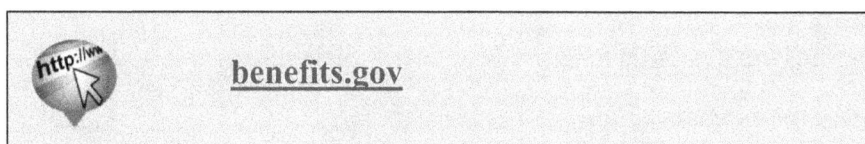

benefits.gov

- Find the **BENEFITS** drop-down menu at the top of the screen and choose:
- **BROWSE BY CATEGORY**—offers a variety of options to choose from based on need
- **BENEFIT FINDER**—completely answer all the questions to see what you qualify for

Contact information by State for Medicare & Medicaid Service Centers

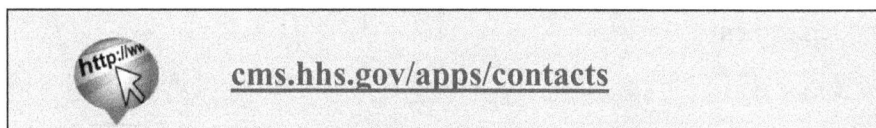

cms.hhs.gov/apps/contacts

Medicaid Programs

Adult Benefits Waiver Programs

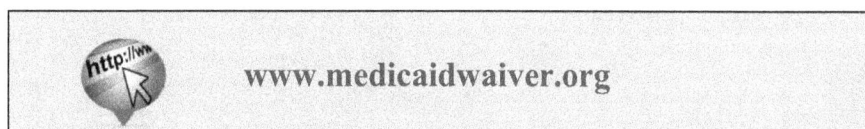

www.medicaidwaiver.org

Select the link for your state from the list located in the center of the page.

- The programs and contact information are provided for each state—call the number to obtain further details regarding the various waiver programs available
- The eligibility criteria is different and more expansive than general Medicaid, therefore *those who do not qualify for general Medicaid, often qualify here*
- Depending on the state, these waiver programs may benefit the elderly, children and young adults, those with brain injuries, HIV or AIDS, and more...

State information includes:

- Which programs are available to assist people with disabilities?
- Who qualifies for assistance?
- Is there a waiting list for services?
- What services are offered and what are the service limitations?
- How do you select a provider?
- How do you become a provider?
- Additional information

Waiver coverage may include:

- Emergency department
- Laboratory & X-ray
- Medical supplies / durable medical equipment
- Mental health service
- Outpatient hospital (low co-pay)
- Pharmacy (low co-pay)
- Physician visits (low co-pay)
- Substance abuse
- Urgent Care Clinic (low co-pay)
- More...

Note from Camille:

This is a VERY important site for you to consider. The Waiver Program alone saved thousands of dollars in products and services that were needed and required while caring for my parents.

Supplemental Nutritional Assistance Program (SNAP)

This is the new name given to the food stamps program as of October 2008.

- SNAP helps low-income families buy the food they need

- Benefits are distributed via a card similar to an ATM card that is accepted at most grocery stores

- **Note**: This the **national** name—your state may have a different name for the program

- Each state has different criteria for eligibility

www.fns.usda.gov/snap/applicant-recipient

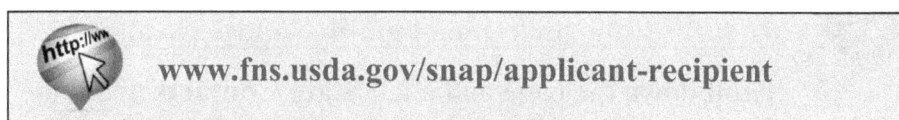

- Select the link **find a local SNAP office** located in the second paragraph

- From the **MAP** that comes up (from either link above) on the **STATE Directory of Resources** page—click the state you desire for all the contact information you will need including the **Program Name, Telephone number(s), State SNAP & EBT information, Website links,** and the **State online applications** link

Note from Camille:

IMPORTANT TIP TO QUALIFY FOR FOOD STAMPS

You may have been told you make too much money to qualify for food stamps—or if you do qualify, the monthly food stamp allowance you are offered may be lower than you hoped.

Here is a tip that is not often shared, and can make a huge difference as to whether you qualify for food assistance or not.

If you are a senior over the age of 60—or if you are disabled (no matter what your age)—you are able to use your outstanding medical bills to help you qualify.

I began to share this information with several individuals who were initially denied food assistance, or received less than the full amount they could actually qualify for—knowing their individual situations and the outstanding medical bills they all possessed.

Most were lower income seniors, and one was a younger disabled adult.

Each of them were able to qualify for the maximum monthly dollar amount offered by their state—simply by using their outstanding medical bills to help them qualify.

NEVER take NO for an answer *when you are told you don't qualify for something. Keep asking questions, or supply them with the answers you now know to tell them.*

The Emergency Food Assistance Program (TEFAP)

TEFAP is a federally funded program that helps low-income families supplement their diet by providing assistance obtaining emergency food. Local organizations are selected to directly distribute food to households, serve meals, or distribute food to other local organizations that perform these functions.

Main website: **www.fns.usda.gov/tefap**

www.fns.usda.gov/tefap/eligibility-and-how-apply

Scroll down the page and click **State Contacts** under the **How to Apply** section area for state contact information.

Family Caregiver Support—State Contact Information

Some states DO pay family caregivers.

- Pay may be limited

- The level of support varies from state to state and can vary within a state

- Also refer to the **CASH & COUNSELING** section (beginning on **page 39**), as they DO pay a cash stipend to family caregivers in most states

Note: *Cash & Counseling programs often use different names in different states. Therefore, it is important to actually CALL the contact number(s) provided for your state, and ask what the program is called. Investigate all the options these programs provide. Please refer to **pages 39 – 42** for details.*

Many states offer:

- Counseling

- Support groups

- Training

- Respite care

All states provide some relief due to the enactment of the **"Family Caregiver Support Program"** in 2000.

---

acl.gov

This is the website for Administration for Community Living

(202) 401-4634 (Direct number)

(800) 677-1116 (to find local resources through Eldercare Locator)

The above website provides ample information on many programs and resources you may need.

To contact someone from your local area:

- From the website, scroll to the bottom of the page
- On the left side under 'Site Support' select **Contact Us**
- Under the 'Phone Numbers Area' select the link **ACL's Regional Offices**
- **Find your state** under the 'Regional Support Centers'
- Call the contact person at the phone number provided and ask about the **"Family Caregiver Support Program"**
  - Ask any specific questions you may have regarding respite care, money available for caregivers, or other questions you wish to inquire about

---

Eldercare Locator:

eldercare.acl.gov to find HELP in your community by **zip code**

Adult Family Care Program

eldercare.org
OR
adultfamilycare.org

(617) 628-2601 (for eldercare.org)

(617) 440-0987 (for adultfamilycare.org)
8 a.m. – 5 p.m. EST (Monday – Friday)

Ask for information on **"Adult Family Care"**

Eldercare.org provides services for Somerville, Cambridge, and the Greater Boston Area of Massachusetts.

- Family Caregivers may receive up to $18,000 per year to provide care that prevents or delays nursing home care

- Person must be:

  - Sick or disabled person 18+ years of age AND

  - Eligible for MassHealth

To find out if other areas in Massachusetts have similar programs, contact **Massachusetts Elders.**

Massachusetts Elders:
(800) 243-4636 or (617) 222-7408

HEALTHCARE CENTERS

Health Resources & Services Administration (HRSA) is the primary *federal* agency for improving access to health care (among other services), with centers to care for you even if you have no health insurance. You generally pay what you can afford based on your income, and some are **FREE!**

There is more information on **FREE** or **low-cost MEDICAL CLINICS** in this Resource Guide (see **pages 136 – 139**). The link below provides information for HRSA Healthcare Centers that may be available.

Health Centers may provide:

- Wellness checkups
- Treatment when you're sick
- Complete pregnancy care
- Immunizations and checkups for children
- Dental care
- Prescription drugs
- Mental healthcare
- Substance abuse care

Health centers are located in most cities and many rural areas.

Find A Health Center:

findahealthcenter.hrsa.gov

- From the website, enter the **number of miles** you are willing to travel
- Enter **city and state** (then select the search icon)—the healthcare centers in your area will appear

STATE, COUNTY & CITY PROGRAMS

Adult Day Care

- Available in almost every city or county

- Adult day centers are generally run by a government entity, or through local charities or religious organizations

- Provide seniors with a safe place to socialize, play cards or games, exercise, or eat a hot meal

- Requirements vary from place to place

- Usually accommodate those who need some supervision—yet not candidates for nursing homes

- Activities vary from facility to facility

- May be a nominal cost involved to participate

- Many are **FREE**

- Call local Office for the Aging (like the Area Agencies on Aging, **page 26**) for more information

Home Chore / Chore Services

Because many of the additional services are run by your **LOCAL** community, please check into these services, **even if you or your loved one do not qualify for your state Medicaid Waiver Program**. You will be surprised at the programs you or your loved one may qualify for and be able to use.

Many municipalities have services—some provided by volunteers—to help seniors and/or physically disabled adults with household chores. **THERE IS NO SINGLE COMPREHENSIVE LIST** of the agencies and organizations that provide these services. You will have to search the **Internet**—contact your **local Area Agency on Aging** (see **page 26**)—or refer to the **Miscellaneous Organizations** section listed in this Resource Guide (beginning on **page 190**) for organizations that offer programs or volunteer help for these services.

Search online for the following terms. Be sure to include the name of your state in your search.

- chore services
- home chore services

- chore services programs
- home chore services programs

SEARCH RESULTS EXAMPLE:

In the address bar of your browser type in:

"Chore services (your state)" or "Chore Services programs (your state)."

Examples:

- "Chore Services Alabama"
- "Chore Services programs Wisconsin"

Every program is different, offering different services with potentially different criteria for qualifying. Be sure to read the full descriptions to see if the service you require is offered. If it's not, check further, as other programs may be available in your area.

The following **EXAMPLES** are descriptions from three Chore Services programs offered in various parts of the country. Note that the first does not offer outdoor work. The second mentions the average number of hours per month they will work for a single client. The third mentions the possibility of pairing the client with a high school student looking to obtain some volunteer hours.

EXAMPLE 1

Services are provided for homeowners who are age 60 and over and / or physically disabled, age 18 and over. Work is performed by volunteer handymen and handywomen who are motivated by the desire to help others in the community. Chore volunteers are not licensed carpenters or electricians. They are homeowners who have the knowledge to perform simple household repairs. Each Chore crew will determine if a particular project is within their expertise.

<u>Minor Plumbing</u>
Repair leaking faucets
Repair leaking toilets
Replace washer hoses

<u>Minor Electrical</u>
Replace outlets
Replace light switches and plugs
Replace or repair doorbells
Replace light bulbs
Replace existing light fixture (if appropriate)

<u>Repair or Replace</u>
Door locks, handles, springs and closers
Filters and batteries

<u>Install</u>
Smoke alarms
Carbon monoxide alarms
Grab bars in bath area
Internal railings
Air conditioners (also remove)
Storm windows / screens (also remove)

What Chore CANNOT Do for You

- Chore is unable to service emergencies.

- Chore does not do major outdoor work, painting, tiling, door or window replacements, work requiring high ladders, heavy lifting, new wiring or appliance repairs.

- Chore does not perform cosmetic repairs or provide interior decorating services.

- Repairs for apartment dwellers are limited to personal items only. (Other repairs are the responsibility of the landlord).

If you need the name of a licensed plumber, electrician or other skilled worker, consult the Internet or the Yellow Pages.

EXAMPLE 2

Volunteer Chore Services (VCS) began in 1981 in response to cuts in services for elders by the state legislature. The program currently works with thousands of elders and adults with disabilities statewide. VCS is committed to helping elders and adults with disabilities remain independent in their own homes through a network of caring community members. The services are provided at no charge and serve as a safety net for those individuals who cannot afford to pay for assistance and do not qualify for other assistance. Volunteers generally provide 2 to 8 hours per month assisting their neighbors depending on their schedules and availability.

Services provided include:

- Housework
- Laundry
- Shopping / errands
- Transportation
- Yard Work
- Respite
- Minor home repairs
- Cooking

- Communications
- Household repairs
- Monitoring
- Wood provision
- Some kinds of personal care
- Protective supervision
- Moving assistance

EXAMPLE 3

The Home Chore Volunteer Program was developed in 1986 to assist frail, limited-income senior adults with basic home chores to help them remain independent and in their own homes. The program has grown to include not only individual volunteers but also groups interested in doing a volunteer project for and with senior adults. The program has also expanded into high schools where students are matched with a senior adult to provide household assistance and friendly visitation throughout the school term.

What Services Might Be Provided?

- Light housework
- Clean floors
- Wash windows
- Laundry
- Take out garbage

- Friendly visitation
- Minor home repairs
- Garden work
- Shovel snow

Do a thorough Internet search for **your city, county, and / or state,** and carefully read the descriptions. You will then know whether the services you seek are offered through the program(s) in your area.

Property Improvement Programs

National Residential Improvement Association:
nria.org

(877) 591-2672 (toll free)
9 a.m. – 6 p.m. EST (Monday – Friday)

The government offers a variety of home improvement programs that may **help pay for necessary home improvements**.

You may qualify for grants, government insured loans, tax credits, discounts, and other special home improvement programs **most consumers are unaware of.**

If you need help determining the types of programs you may qualify for:

- Select the **Application** tab on the menu at the top of the homepage

- Complete the brief questionnaire

- Select the **Submit** button and an NRIA Program Specialist will contact you to help determine which programs you may be eligible for

  - The specialist will also point you in the right direction to help get things started

- You can also jump ahead a bit (if you are curious) and select the **Programs** tab (also at the top of the homepage) to see all the programs offered in your state

- Most consumers have no idea these programs even exist, so be sure to speak to an NRIA Program Specialist

- Write down any questions you may wish to ask

- Don't forget make a copy of the checklist at the end of this section to write notes during the call

All services provided by NRIA are FREE to consumers.

Another alternative is to call your local **COUNTY** and ask for **"Property Improvement Programs."**

EXAMPLE of a Property Improvement Loan in Michigan

Eligibility:

- Gross household income up to $105,700—home must be primary residence of borrower

- Minimum 620 credit score required to qualify for low interest loan—loan amount & interest will vary based on income—up to 20 years to repay

- Larger loan amounts require a minimum credit score of 660

Improvements that may be eligible to qualify for loan:

- Insulation
- Windows
- Doors
- Plumbing

- Septic tanks
- Roof replacement
- Air conditioner and more…

Financial Hardship Property Tax Exemptions

These are **LOCAL MUNICIPAL** programs.

Many municipalities have programs to help **seniors** and **physically disabled** adults pay their property taxes. There are also exemptions for **veterans**, **hardships**, and others. Always check, as there are multiple avenues to pursue that you may qualify for. Each state and city is different, so you must check your individual state and city.

THERE IS NO SINGLE COMPREHENSIVE LIST of the agencies that provide this help. You will have to search the Internet or contact your city / town / or village for more information. You may include the name of your **city / town / village** in your search.

- In the address bar of your browser type in:

  - **"Residential Property Tax Exemptions (your state)"**

  - **"Residential Property Tax Exemptions (your city and state)"**

  - **"Financial Hardship Residential Property Tax Exemptions (your state)"**

OR

- **"Financial Hardship Residential Property Tax Exemptions (your city and state)"**

Examples:

- "Residential Property Tax Exemptions California"

- "Residential Property Tax Exemptions Boulder, Colorado"

- "Financial Hardship Residential Property Tax Exemptions Parma, Ohio"

- You *may* be eligible to receive an exemption on your property taxes

- **Criteria:**

  - You must meet federal poverty income standards OR

  - You are a disabled veteran

    OR

  - You are in a hardship situation

  - **For veterans**: I was able to locate a website that has all the qualifications and criteria for each individual state in one convenient location. Scroll down the page and **select your state** for more information.

For veterans:

www.veteransunited.com/futurehomeowners/veteran-property-tax-exemptions-by-state

---

File your claim with the CITY / TOWN / VILLAGE Supervisor or Board of Review.

You may have to ASK for these exemptions, as they may not be offered to you voluntarily.

Contact your **CITY / TOWN / VILLAGE** for program and eligibility information.

Homestead Property Tax Credit

These are **STATE** programs through which **seniors** and **other individuals** may qualify to receive property tax credits.

THERE IS NO SINGLE COMPREHENSIVE LIST of the agencies that provide these tax credits. You will have to search the Internet or contact your state for more information. Be sure to include the name of your state in your search.

- In the address bar of your browser type in: **"Homestead Property Tax Credits (your state)"**

Examples:

- "Homestead Property Tax Credits Florida"
- "Homestead Property Tax Credits Michigan"

You may have to ASK for these homestead property tax credits, as they may not be offered to you voluntarily.

EXAMPLE for Michigan

- Seniors (age 65 by December 31st of the tax year), may be eligible to receive property tax credits

- May file up to four years from the annual date

- Maximum amount $1,500 credit per year

- Property tax credit received by filing form MI-1040CR

Contact your **STATE** for program and eligibility information.

Family Services Senior Homemaking & Respite Care Programs

These may be **COUNTY** or **STATE** programs.

Many counties and states have services to help **seniors** and / or **physically disabled adults** with homemaking and respite care.

If searching the Internet, be sure to include the name of your state in your search.

- Type **"Respite Care Programs (your state or county and state)"** into the address bar of your browser—simply substitute the state you are searching for

Example:

- "Respite Care Programs DuPage County, IL"

EXAMPLE: New Jersey Statewide Respite Care Program

The NJ Statewide Respite Care Program has been operational since April of 1988. This program provides respite care services for elderly and functionally impaired persons age 18 and older to relieve their unpaid caregivers of stress arising from the responsibility of providing daily care. A secondary goal of the program is to provide the support necessary to help families avoid making nursing home placement of their relatives.

Services available under the Statewide Respite Care Program include:

- Companions
- Homemaker / home health aides (on an hourly or overnight basis)
- Medical or social adult day care
- Camperships

- Private duty nursing service
- Temporary care in licensed medical facilities
- Caregiver-directed option

> To reach the Statewide Respite Care Program in your county, call Aging & Disability Resource Connection (ADRC):
>
> (877) 222-3737

Please refer to: **RESPITECARE** section **(page 156)**; **MISCELLANEOUS ORGANIZATIONS** section **(page 190)** and scroll through the list; and **AREA AGENCIES ON AGING** section **(page 26)** to find local programs] of this Resource Guide to find more programs and organizations offering respite care.

Contact your **COUNTY or STATE** for program and eligibility information.

Minor Home Repairs

These are generally **CITY** programs.

Many municipalities have services to **help seniors**, **physically disabled adults**, and **low-income individuals** with minor home repairs. Each city and county is different with different eligibility and income requirements.

See example on next page.

EXAMPLE: Phoenix Community Action Program

Three multipurpose Family Services Centers are located throughout the city and provide a broad range of services to promote self-sufficiency for adults and families. Services may include:

Case Management

- Caseworkers help adult individuals and families resolve social service problems and assist them in achieving self-sufficiency.

- Examples of assistance include budgeting, social and life-skills development, counseling and direct services.

Emergency Financial Assistance

- This includes rental and utility assistance in crisis situations. Other emergency services are provided as center resources allow.

Assistance may include (examples):

- financial assistance

- information on senior programs and resources

- minor home repairs

- senior discount programs

- nutritional resources

- transportation services

To access senior services, call the Senior Services Intake line at:
(602) 262-6631

Or the City of Phoenix general information line at:
(602) 262-6011
8 a.m. – 4:30 p.m. (Monday – Friday). They will direct you to the closest Family Service Center.

Many of these services are provided through grants or government programs. There are also volunteer organizations that will help and assist seniors with minor home repairs. Many of these programs are **FREE**.

In the address bar of your browser type in **your state** or **city and state** as follows:

- **"Minor Home Repair Assistance Programs (your state)"**

- **"Minor Home Repair Assistance Programs (your city and state)"**

Examples:

- "Minor Home Repair Assistance Programs Ohio"

- "Minor Home Repair Assistance Programs Ft. Lauderdale, FL"

A variety of programs should come up for you to choose from.

Please also refer to:

MISCELLANEOUS section (page 190) for volunteer programs, and 'local'

Home Chore & Chore Services (page 55)

Contact your **CITY / TOWN / VILLAGE** for program availability and eligibility information.

TELEPHONE TECHNIQUES

When calling your local area resource numbers, it may be wise to follow a few guidelines that will prove helpful. These techniques may encourage the person you are speaking with to give all the necessary information you are requesting, without becoming impatient with your list of questions. There is no single formula for success. However, *persistence* usually prevails when all else fails.

SUGGESTIONS:

Be prepared

- Have the agency name, telephone number, and your questions written down *before* you make the call

- Have several pens and a pad of paper available (or use the checklists provided)

- Schedule at least 30 minutes to devote to the telephone call

- Make sure you are rested before you call

- Write down the name of the person you speak with

  - If the person appears helpful, you should be able to contact them again in the future should you need clarification or further help

  - If they are not particularly knowledgeable or helpful, you may want to speak to someone else, or a supervisor, the next time you call

Ask open-ended questions

- Ask questions that require at least a one-sentence response, as opposed to questions that simply have 'yes' or 'no' answers

- This will encourage the person you are speaking with to give more information

Be cordial, yet persistent

- Make sure you are in a good mood when you call
- As the saying goes: "You catch more bees with honey than with vinegar!"
- Your vocal tone, inflection, and mood will come across on the telephone, so try to start with a smile
- People are more likely to help someone who is pleasant than someone who is cranky or demanding
- Compliment the person—tell them you appreciate their helpfulness, knowledge, and / or understanding

Have a family member or friend call if you are:

- Not the most diplomatic person
- Exhausted
- Overwhelmed by your caregiving activities and responsibilities
- Running into a roadblock

CHECKLISTS FOR GOVERNMENT RESOURCES

MEDICARE

Note: *Author grants permission for you to make copies of this checklist for your future needs and as your information changes.*

http://	ssa.gov (Social Security) or medicare.gov (Medicare)
📱	(800) 772-1213 or (800) 325-0778 TTY
	(800) 633-4227 or (877) 486-2048 TTY (Medicare)

CONTACT PERSON	
Date to apply:	
Dates called:	

MEDICARE PART D

Note: Author grants permission for you to make copies of this checklist for your future needs and as your information changes.

Make a list of all your medications, the strength of the medication, and how often you them.

MEDICATION	STRENGTH (Dose)	FREQUENCY (How often it's taken)	#Tablets / Vials Used per Month

Check with local pharmacies about drug prices, including generics. Don't forget to also check the discount drug cards listed in the prescription section of this book.

MEDICAID

WAIVER LOCAL AREA PROGRAM

Note: *Author grants permission for you to make copies of this checklist for your future needs and as your information changes.*

NAME of LOCAL PROGRAM	
CONTACT PERSON	
Dates called:	
My state does / does not have a "Cash & Counseling" program.	☐ DOES HAVE ☐ DOES NOT HAVE *Please see **pages 39 – 42** for details.*

RESPITE CARE PROGRAM

Note: *Author grants permission for you to make copies of this checklist for your future needs and as your information changes.*

NAME of LOCAL PROGRAM	
📱	
🌐	
CONTACT PERSON	
Dates called:	

CHORE SERVICES PROGRAM

Note: *Author grants permission for you to make copies of this checklist for your future needs and as your information changes.*

NAME of LOCAL PROGRAM	
📱	
http://w	
CONTACT PERSON	
Dates called:	
PRICES	$ $ $

MEDICARE SAVINGS PROGRAM

Note: *Author grants permission for you to make copies of this checklist for your future needs and as your information changes.*

📱	
http://	
CONTACT PERSON	
Dates called:	

PRESCRIPTION ASSISTANCE PROGRAM

Note: *Author grants permission for you to make copies of this checklist for your future needs and as your information changes.*

NAME of LOCAL PROGRAM	
CONTACT PERSON	
Dates called:	

ADULT BENEFITS WAIVER PROGRAM

Note: *Author grants permission for you to make copies of this checklist for your future needs and as your information changes.*

CONTACT PERSON	
Dates called:	

SUPPLEMENTAL NUTRITION ASSISTANCE PROGRAM (SNAP)
also known as "Food Stamps"

Note: *Author grants permission for you to make copies of this checklist for your future needs and as your information changes.*

NAME of LOCAL PROGRAM	
CONTACT PERSON	
Dates called:	

STATE PROGRAMS

Note: *Author grants permission for you to make copies of this checklist for your future needs and as your information changes.*

NAME of PROGRAM	NAME of PROGRAM
CONTACT PERSON	**CONTACT PERSON**
Dates called: _____ _____	Dates called: _____ _____

STATE PROGRAMS

Note: *Author grants permission for you to make copies of this checklist for your future needs and as your information changes.*

NAME of PROGRAM	NAME of PROGRAM
CONTACT PERSON	**CONTACT PERSON**
Dates called: _____ _____	Dates called: _____ _____

COUNTY PROGRAMS

Note: *Author grants permission for you to make copies of this checklist for your future needs and as your information changes.*

NAME of PROGRAM	NAME of PROGRAM
CONTACT PERSON	CONTACT PERSON
Dates called: _____ _____	Dates called: _____ _____

COUNTY PROGRAMS

Note: *Author grants permission for you to make copies of this checklist for your future needs and as your information changes.*

NAME of PROGRAM	NAME of PROGRAM
CONTACT PERSON	CONTACT PERSON
Dates called: _____	Dates called: _____

CITY / TOWN / VILLAGE PROGRAMS

Note: *Author grants permission for you to make copies of this checklist for your future needs and as your information changes.*

NAME of PROGRAM	NAME of PROGRAM
CONTACT PERSON	CONTACT PERSON
Dates called: _____	Dates called: _____

CITY / TOWN / VILLAGE PROGRAMS

Note: *Author grants permission for you to make copies of this checklist for your future needs and as your information changes.*

NAME of PROGRAM	NAME of PROGRAM
CONTACT PERSON	**CONTACT PERSON**
Dates called: _____ _____	**Dates called:** _____ _____

BENEFICIAL RESOURCES

RESOURCES BY SERVICE

"Seek and you shall find.
Knock and the door will be opened unto you."

—Jesus of Nazareth

CLOTHING

Salvation Army

- **Low-cost** clothing—often new with price tags still on them
- Price stickers on all items in store are color-coded
    - Each week, a designated color sticker entitles 50% off final price
    - In some states—on Friday and Saturday of that same week—all clothes with the weekly color sticker are priced five items for $5
- Every state has their own system offering sale item discounts
    - Please check the discount policies of your local Salvation Army store(s)
- Senior discounts available
    - Day of week and percent discounted vary by state (often 30%)
- Also offers deep discounts on a variety of miscellaneous household items and books

---

salvationarmyusa.org

From Homepage:
In the upper right-hand corner

- Enter **zip code** in box provided
- Will provide **contact information** for a Salvation Army in your area

---

(800) SAL-ARMY (main number)

(800) 725-2769

Goodwill

- **Low-cost** clothing in very good to excellent condition—sometimes new

- Senior discounts available

  - Day of week may vary

  - Percent discounted also varies by state (generally 25%)

- 50% discount on everything in the store on a designated day—often every other Saturday—or during the week with designated weekly colored-coded sticker

  - Check for specifics in your area

- Also offers deep **discounts** on a variety of miscellaneous household items and books

---

goodwill.org

From Homepage:

Hover over the **SHOP** tab and select **Find a Store** from the dropdown menu to find your nearest Goodwill location

---

(800) GOODWILL (main number)

(800) 466-3945

---

*Local churches and community centers also offer **FREE** clothing if you cannot afford to pay.*

EYE / VISION CARE

Free Eyeglasses

Lions Club

World's largest service club organization—primary focus is to help prevent blindness all over the world.

- Provide **FREE** eyeglasses and eye exam to those who qualify
  - Usually hardship cases—approved on a case-by-case basis
- Other programs are also available including feeding the hungry, and helping those in need
- Contact your **local** Lions Club for more details on programs, including Special Olympics

http://	lionsclubs.org
📱	(630) 571-5466
✉ MAIL	Lions Clubs International Headquarters 300 W. 22nd Street Oak Brook, IL 60523-8842

Discounted Eyeglasses

Dollar Stores

- May obtain non-prescription reading glasses for $1 at most any local 'Dollar Store' in your area
- Many varieties to choose from—often known brands
- In a pinch, when you are low on cash, or simply because it is a personal choice—a viable alternative to prescription readers

$39 Eyeglasses (this is the name of the company)

- Single-lens eyeglasses from $39—bifocals from $79

- 100% quality guarantee

- Included **FREE**:

  - Light and thin prescription lenses

  - Scratch-resistant coating

  - Hard carrying case

  - Cleaning cloth

  - 100% UV protection

  - Shipping on orders over $99

39dollarglasses.com

(800) 672-6304

(631) 557-0613

9 a.m.—5 p.m. EST

America's Best

- Local stores in many areas of the country

- Eyeglass company providing discounted eye exams and lenses

  - Single-lens—two pair for $69.95 & **FREE** eye exam

  - Bifocals—two pair for $99.95 & **FREE** eye exam

---

americasbest.com

To **FIND A STORE** near you, enter **zip code** or **city and state** in the search box.

In-store orders:
(800) 411-1162
9 a.m. – 6 p.m. EST (Monday – Friday)

Online orders:

(800) 999-4758
9 a.m. – 8 p.m. EST (Monday – Friday)
9 a.m. – 5:30 p.m. EST (Saturday)

EyeBuyDirect.com

- Single-lens eyeglasses from $6.95—bifocals add $29—progressive lenses add $39

- Unconditional guarantee

  - Refund for any reason within 14 days after receiving frames, less S&H

  - Does not apply to designer and sport frames

- 30% student discount

- Has an 'Eye Try' area:

  - Upload your photo and try on the frames

  - Faces of models also available to try on the frames

- Shipping & Handling: $5.95 per pair

- Included **FREE**:

  - Anti-scratch coating

  - Hard carrying case

  - Cleaning cloth

  - Shipping on orders over $99

- May offer coupons occasionally

- Has "Deal of the Week" with up to 30% discount

http://	**eyebuydirect.com**
	(855) 393-2891 9 a.m. – Midnight EST (Monday – Friday) 9 a.m. – 6 p.m. EST (Saturday and Sunday)

Zenni Optical

- Single-lens eyeglasses from $6.95—bifocals from $17—progressives from $27.95
- Included **FREE**:
  - Anti-scratch coat
  - Full UV protection
  - Hard carrying case, microfiber cloth
  - Has area to download your picture to try on the frames
  - Guarantee
- Shipping & Handling: $4.95 per order (no matter how large an order you place)

http://	**zennioptical.com**
	(800) 211-2105 5 a.m.—9 p.m. PST
@	**service@zennioptical.com**

DENTAL SERVICES (FREE or Discounted)

National Dental Lifeline Network

- Provides **FREE** dental services for the **elderly, handicapped**, or **medically at risk** who cannot afford dental treatment or obtain public aid
- Also make **house calls** for those unable to travel to dentists' offices
  - This service provided in Metro Chicago and Colorado at this time

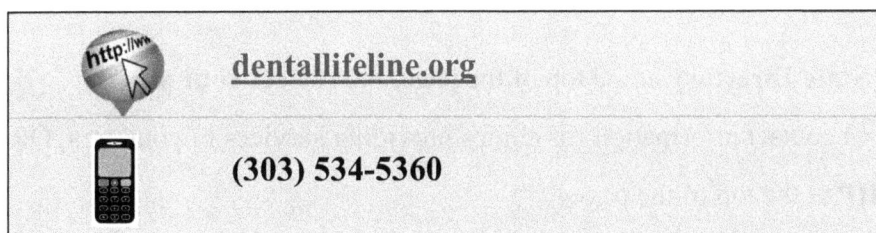

dentallifeline.org

(303) 534-5360

From the website select the link that says **STATE PROGRAMS** (top of page)

- **Map** of United States will appear—**Select your state**
  - Contact information and eligibility requirements will come up
  - Submit application, or call the number directly if you have questions

DentalPlans.com

- Nationwide program that offers many discount dental plans
  - These are **discounted** dental plans, not dental insurance
  - Yearly premiums are far less expensive than traditional dental plans
  - May offer vision, hearing, prescription **discounts**, cosmetic dental (depends on plan)

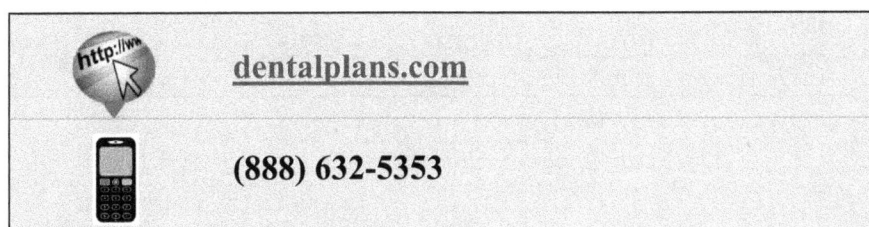

dentalplans.com

(888) 632-5353

FREE-Dentistry.com

- Provides **FREE** or **low-cost** dental healthcare to qualifying individuals who are disabled, **elderly, medically compromised, children**, and **low-income**—through public and private programs

- Website offers many other options including multiple services, articles, video information, tutorials, and specific information regarding your teeth

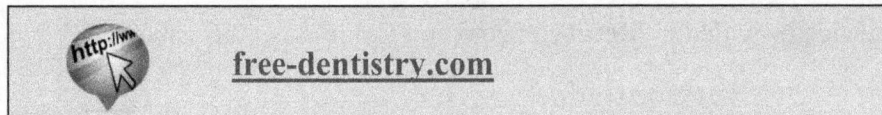

> **free-dentistry.com**

- Select the **State Directory** at the top of the page, then **select your state**

  - Provides contact information for clinics providing services in your area, OR

- Select **CHIP** at the top of the page

  - Provides **low-cost** health insurance for children in families who do not qualify for Medicaid and cannot afford private health insurance

Health Resources and Services Administration (HRSA)

- Supports federally funded community health centers nationwide that provide **FREE**, **reduced-cost** or **low-cost** health services—including dental services

  - **FREE** dental care

  - **FREE** dental services

  - **FREE** dental clinics

  - And much more...

  - Enter your **zip code** in the search area—a list of health clinics that are geographically close to you will appear

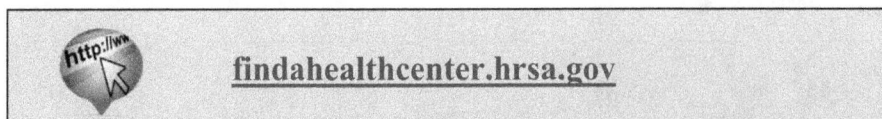

> **findahealthcenter.hrsa.gov**

Examples of several programs available in Michigan:

Donated Dental Services (DDS)

- Program of the Michigan Dental Association and the National Foundation of Dentistry for the Disabled, Medically at Risk, or Elderly—with no other way to pay

  - Generally, service provided **FREE**

  - May ask for partial payment if you can afford it

  - Must fill out application to be seen

  - May often wait up to a year for services

  - Services nine counties in the state of Michigan

(800) 850-5913

DMC Dental Clinic

- Located in Detroit Receiving Hospital
- 50% price reduction or sliding scale based on income
- No insurance necessary to be seen

(313) 745-1977 and (313) 745-3000

Detroit Area Dental Schools providing Discounted Dental Services:

University of Detroit Dental School
(313) 494-6700

University of Michigan Dental School
(888) 707-2500 or **(734) 763-6933**

These services are provided by dental students and supervised by licensed dentists.

Every state is different, so check the dental schools in your area for the cost of services.

To find a Donated Dental Services Program in your state:

- Type **"Donated Dental Services (your state)"** in the address bar of your browser
  - **Example:** "Donated Dental Services Mississippi"
  - **Example:** "Donated Dental Services Oregon"
  - **Select the link for your state**—the contact information should be readily available for you

SPECIAL ADDITIONAL RESOURCES FOR THOSE WITH DISABILITIES and SPECIAL NEEDS

The websites listed below provide **FREE** materials, resources, and service animals for those with disabilities. ***Please refer to bottom of page 132 for many additional discounts.***

For the Blind

Braille Books

- **American Action Fund for Blind Children and Adults**
  - Provides **FREE** Braille Books Program

http://	**www.actionfund.org/FREE-braille-books**
📱	(410) 659-9315, ext. 1
@	**actionfund@actionfund.org**

- **Braille Institute**
  - Provides **FREE** books for children in Braille

http://	**www.brailleinstitute.org/special-collection**
📱	**(323) 906-3104** or **(800) BRAILLE (272-4553)** 8:30 a.m. – 5p.m. PST (Monday – Friday)
@	**specialcollection@brailleinstitute.org**

- **Seedlings**
  - Provides **two FREE** Braille books per year for children, under the "Book Angel Program"

http://	**http://www.seedlings.org/special.php**
📱	(734) 427-8552 or (800) 777-8552 9 a.m. – 5 p.m. EST
@	info@seedlings.org

- **WonderBaby.org**
  - Provides **FREE**, paid, and downloadable Braille books from various resources
  - May also download musical scores, magazines, and books from Web-Braille

http://	**www.wonderbaby.org/articles/best-braille-childrens-book-resources-internet**
📱	No phone number available.
@	help@wonderbaby.org

Leader Dogs for the Blind

- Located in Rochester, Michigan
- Provide **FREE** leader dogs for the blind
- Founded by several Lions Club members in 1939
- In addition to guide dog training, programs available in:
  - Orientation and mobility training

- GPS training

- Seminars for orientation and mobility professionals

- Deaf-Blind Guide Dog Program

  o These are NOT hearing dogs

  o Trained on hand signals only

- Hover over the **RESOURCES** tab at the top of the page and select **PEOPLE WHO ARE BLIND** from the dropdown menu

  - This link provides many helpful and useful resources (including literature) to view

http://w	**leaderdog.org** May email directly by clicking the **CONTACT US** link at the bottom of the page • Fill out the required information
📱	(888) 777-5332 (248) 651-9011
@	**leaderdog@leaderdog.org**

For the Hearing Impaired

Hearing Aids

Hearing loss is extremely prevalent among the elderly. Hearing aid devices can be one of the largest out-of-pocket expenses a hearing impaired person can have—often ranging upward to $4,000+ per device.

It is only recently that discounts on hearing devices have become more affordable to the average person through various discount houses, websites, and the organizations that sell them.

Although Medicare does not generally cover the cost of these devices, some Medicare Advantage plans and alternate healthcare plans do cover at least a part of the cost—even if purchased through a discount facility.

If you do not have an Advantage plan or other healthcare plan, you will pay 20% of the approved amount of the doctor visit or hearing test—excluding the cost of the hearing aid itself.

For this reason, compare your options from various discount hearing aid companies so you are not overpaying. Your out-of-pocket cost will be a small portion of the original retail cost for these products, and you can easily save up to 80%.

Being a member of a Medicare Advantage plan (including those from AARP), often helps with costs—as you will receive even larger **discounts** from many of the following companies.

- **hi Health Innovations**

  - Deeply discounted hearing aids available

  - Locations in various states provided

  > **hiHealthInnovations.com**
  >
  > (855) 523-9355

  - Select the **Locations** tab at the top of page

    o Find your state for more contact information and details

  - To obtain hearing aids from this company:

    o Schedule an appointment to test your hearing by calling **(855) 523-9355**

    OR

    o Submit results of most recent hearing test if obtained within the past year

    o Hover over the **Hearing Aids** tab at the top of the page

    o From the dropdown menu select **How to Order**

      • Specific details are provided

      • Follow the instructions

  - Home delivery option available versus picking up at purchase location

  - 70-Day return policy versus 30-45 day trial through most retailers or traditional dispensers (no restocking fee)

  - **FREE** hearing aid adjustments—if needed

- Protection Plan available if device is lost or damaged

- Additional **discounts** through Medicare Advantage plans like

  o AARP Complete

  o AARP MedicareRx

  o United Healthcare

- **Veterans** may apply and qualify through VA as follows:

  o *In person* at any VA Medical Office or Clinic

  o *Online* by filling out **Form 10-10EZ**

  o *Through the mail* by completing **Form 10-10EZ** and mailing it to the Medical Center of your choice

- **Veterans** who do not qualify for coverage (including spouses)—receive $100 additional discount on purchase

- Private insurance and other healthcare plans *may* pay for some of the charges

- Straight Medicare does not pay for hearing aids

  o You pay 20% of the doctor office Medicare approved amount

  o Part B deductible applies

- From dropdown menu at the top of the page under **How to Order**

  o Select the link that says **Medicare & Insurance Coverage**

  o Scroll down the page to view various programs (including the VA) that help pay for costs

  o Select the highlighted links in various sections for more information

- Price: From $799 and up

- **Discount Hearing Aids of America**

  - Veteran owned

  - Discounted hearing aids available from a variety of name-brand manufacturers

  - Reconditioned hearing aids available to further reduce cost

  - Prior generation models available from name-brand manufacturers

  - No insurance included—may be purchased from third-party vendors

  - Six month warranty—12-month warranty if two units purchased

  - Styles available:

- o Analog
- o Basic
- o Standard digital
- o Advanced digital
- o Premium
- ▪ Price: From $495 reconditioned, from $1,095 new

DiscountHearingAidsOfAmerica.com

(954) 380-9290
(888) 243-2765, (888) 2-HEAR-OK
(954) 628-5210 Fax

info@DiscountHearingAidsOfAmerica.com

- • **Lions Club FREE Hearing Aids Program**

The Lions Club Hearing Aid Recycling Program (HARP) will distribute refurbish donated hearing aids to individuals with low income.

- ▪ Contact Lions Club International to obtain contact information to your local Lions Club
  - o Ask your local Lions Club how to obtain a **FREE** hearing aid from their HARP program

LionsClubs.org

Lions Club International

(630) 571-5466
(ask for contact information to local Lions Club)

CaptionCall

- **FREE** CaptionCall phone for those with professional certification of hearing loss
- CaptionCall Mobile also available for iPad
- **FREE** installation, training, ongoing customer support
- May use live operator who captions what the other party is saying
- Captions sent to your CaptionCall phone or iPad to read
- Cost per minute calls are paid by a federally administrated fund
  - No cost to qualified individuals
- To apply:
  - Select the **Order Now** tab at the top of the page and fill out requested information

AND

  - Have your health care professional select the **How to Certify a Patient** tab at the top of the page and fill out the required information
  - Patient must obtain written certification from hearing-care or healthcare professional stating they have hearing loss and need CaptionCall to help communicate effectively by phone
    - Needs to be done before approval for a CaptionCall phone or CaptionCall Mobile

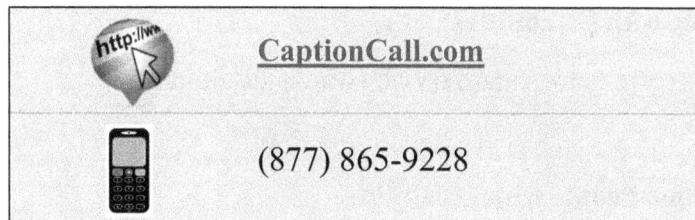

http://ww	**CaptionCall.com**
	(877) 865-9228

Rare Diseases

National Organization for Rare Diseases (NORD)

raredeiseases.org

(203) 744-0100 (National Headquarters - Danbury, CT)
(202) 588-5700 (Washington, DC Office)

Once on the website, select the tab at the top that says **FOR PATIENTS AND FAMILIES**

- Select the link that says **Patient and Caregiver Resource Center**, then scroll all the way down the page and select the link that says **Resources & FAQs**

- This area will provide answers to many of the questions you may have, as well as resources you will be able to contact

- Some of the information obtained from this site includes (and not limited to):

Organizations for People with Disabilities

- Provides a list of organizations that service various disabilities

Resources and Services for People with Disabilities

- Provides a list of services and resources regarding:
  - Wheelchairs
  - Dental clinics for the handicapped and disabled
  - Rehabilitation
  - Jobs
  - Health Resources
  - More...

Resources for Children with Disabilities and Special Needs

- Provides a list of resources for:

  - Families of disabled children

  - Disabled Children's Relief Fund

  - Healthcare for disabled children

  - Parents of disabled children helping other parents with disabled children

  - More...

Other Resources and Tools

- Under the **For Patient and Family** tab, you will find additional information on:

  1. Health Insurance and Medicare / Medicaid Information

  2. Information on Newborn Screening, Genetics, and Lab Testing

  3. Information on Clinical Trials and Research

  4. Resources for People with Disabilities and Special Needs

  5. Government Resources and Other Sites of Interest

  6. Resources from NORD Partners and Resources to Find a Physician

  7. Medical Assistance and much more...

Social Security Benefits For The Disabled

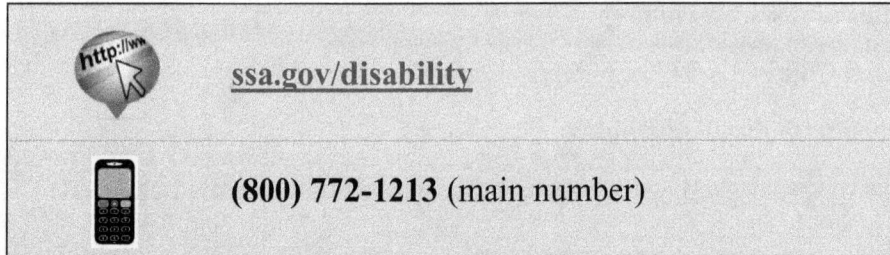

ssa.gov/disability

(800) 772-1213 (main number)

This link provides all the information needed to apply for social security disability including:

- How to apply for benefits
- Obtaining benefits
- Health insurance
- Information about the program
- Frequently asked questions

Children with Disabilities

A disabled child who survives the death of both parents may receive a **"Special Lump-Sum Death Payment"** of **$255** from Social Security. In addition, they may quality for **"Social Security Survivor Benefits"** as well.

Please refer to:
FUNERALS Section of this Resource Guide (page 117) for more details

Please refer to:
LICENSE PLATES section (page 129) for reduced-fee license plates and ASKING for discounts (page 132)

Please refer to
THERAPY ANIMALS / SERVICE ANIMALS section (page 161) as these animals also service the physically and emotionally disabled

Most of the service animals (primarily dogs) are FREE to those who qualify. All you have to do is apply for them. There is often a waiting list, so apply early. You can always cancel if you find you no longer need or want animal assistance.

ENERGY ASSISTANCE

Low Income Home Energy Assistance Program (LIHEAP)

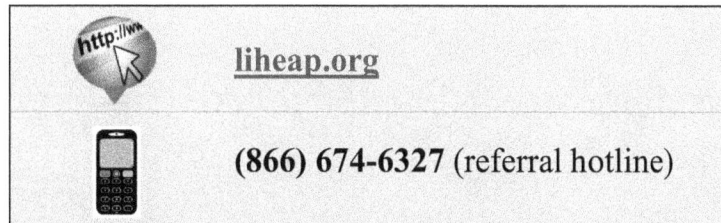

liheap.org

(866) 674-6327 (referral hotline)

- Select **FIND HELP** at the very bottom of the page
- Select **FIND LOCAL HELP**
- Select **Search by State**
- **Find your state** from the dropdown box—select it—**find your county** and select **Search**
- If you are unable to obtain the state contact information, call the **National Energy Assistance Referral Hotline** at:

    (866) 674-6327

After making contact, ask about the programs listed below.

Although each state may vary slightly, the programs available are very similar.

Utility Assistance

- Provides **Home Heating Credits** to help with the heating of the home—each state has its own qualifications
- State Emergency Relief (SER)
  - For individuals who have an emergency that threatens their health or safety

Weatherization Assistance Program

- **County** program
- No age requirement

- **FREE** to those who qualify
- Income eligibility qualifications will vary from county to county within your state
- Can provide
  - New roof
  - New windows / window repair
  - Caulking
  - Other services related to weatherization

Salvation Army

- Provides utility assistance to get through a crisis—contact your local center
- Some states have a local Salvation Army center locator link on the website, under the charitable section
- Provides relief and elderly services
- Salvation Army offers **FREE** furniture and clothing to victims of disasters areas
- Salvation Army also provides **low-cost** furniture, household items, books and more...

> **salvationarmyusa.org**
>
> From Homepage:
> - In the upper right-hand corner
> - Enter **zip code** in box provided for Salvation Army locations in your area
>
> **(800) SAL-ARMY** (main number)
>
> **(800) 725-2769**
> 9 a.m. – 5 p.m. EST (Monday – Friday)

Contact your individual state and county (using the directions above) to find information regarding the programs listed.

FOOD ASSISTANCE

Food assistance is often necessary in many American households. Whether the need arises from a job loss, low income, or other necessary expenses—food shelters, food banks, and a variety of other organizations will provide **FREE food assistance to those who are hungry**.

Feeding America

- Through local and national programs, Feeding America is able to provide **FREE** fresh nutritious food **to Americans facing hunger challenges**

- Donations provide food to people in need through food pantries, soup kitchens, youth programs, senior centers, and emergency shelters

feedingamerica.org

From Homepage:

- Select **Find a Food Bank**

- Under **Find Your Local Food Bank** type in your **zip code**

- Select "**Go**" to find food banks in your area

Meals on Wheels

- Delivers **meals to homebound seniors** who are unable to obtain or prepare food their own food

- **FREE** meals to those who qualify

Eligibility:

- Age 60+

- Homebound or unable to leave home

- Physically or emotionally unable to prepare full meals

- Small donation is suggested for the meal *if* the person is able to contribute

- All donations go back into the program to help provide meals

- Other services may also be available, depending on your state

---

mealsonwheelsamerica.org

(703) 548-5558
9 a.m. – 5:30 p.m. EST (Monday – Friday)

(888) 998-6325 (toll free)

Call the above number(s) to be directed to the Meals on Wheels program in your area.
or
Select the **FIND MEALS** tab at top of page and enter your **zip code** in the **Search by Zip Code** box for a local program in your area.

If you would like to donate your time delivering meals or money to support the program, call the number above to be connected with a coordinator.

Salvation Army

- Provides food for those in need throughout the year— volunteers deliver meals & groceries on Thanksgiving, Christmas, & Easter, to homebound or struggling families

- Some locations offer a hot lunch program for seniors…and many, many other services

---

salvationarmyusa.org

From Homepage:
In the upper right-hand corner

- Enter **zip code** in box provided

- Will provide **contact information** for a Salvation Army in your area

---

(800) SAL-ARMY (main number)

(800) 725-2769

9 a.m.—5p.m. EST (Monday – Friday)

Seniors Farmers' Market Nutrition Program (SFMNP)

- Federal program that provides **low-income seniors** coupons to exchange at farmers markets, roadside stands, and community supported agriculture programs for fresh fruits and vegetables

- Exchange coupons for fresh, locally grown fruits and vegetables (also honey and herbs)

- Available in all 50 states

Eligibility:

- Age 60+

- Income no more than 185% of federal poverty income guidelines

www.fns.usda.gov/

From the website:

- Select **Programs** at the top of page

- From the dropdown menu select **Senior Farmers' Market Nutrition Program**

- Scroll down the page and select the link **State Agency Contacts**

- **Select your state** from the dropdown menu

- All contact information is provided

Supplemental Nutritional Assistance Program (SNAP)

- This is the new name for the Federal Food Stamp Program as of October 2008

- Helps **low-income** families buy the food they need

- SNAP is the national name—your state may have a different name for the program
    - Each state has different criteria for eligibility
- Benefits distributed via an ATM-type card that is accepted at most grocery stores
- Visit the website to apply for benefits or to find your local office

www.fns.usda.gov/snap/applicant-recipient

- In the second paragraph, select the link **"find a local SNAP office"**
    - **Map** of United States appears—**select your state**
    - Hotline number provided
    - Links also provided for online application and local SNAP office

Note from Camille:

IMPORTANT TIP TO QUALIFY FOR FOOD STAMPS

You may have been told you make too much money to qualify for food stamps—or if you do qualify, the monthly food stamp allowance you are offered may be lower than you hoped.

Here is a tip that is not often shared, and can make a huge difference as to whether you qualify for food assistance or not.

If you are a senior over the age of 60—or if you are disabled (no matter what your age)—you are able to use your outstanding medical bills to help you qualify.

I began to share this information with several individuals who were initially denied food assistance, or received less than the full amount they could actually qualify for—knowing their individual situations and the outstanding medical bills they all possessed.

Most were lower income seniors, and one was a younger disabled adult.

All of them were able to qualify for the maximum monthly dollar amount offered by their state—simply by using their outstanding medical bills to help them qualify.

NEVER take NO for an answer *when you are told you don't qualify for something. Keep asking questions, or supply them with the answers you now know to tell them.*

USDA National Hunger Hotline

- Provides callers with contact information for local food pantries or food stamp offices regarding **FREE** food

(866) 3-HUNGRY or (866) 348-6479

(877) 8-HAMBRE or (877) 842-6273 (for Spanish)
7 a.m. – 10 p.m. EST

211

Your local "**211**" is one of your primary resources when any form of community assistance is needed. Some possible examples include (and not limited to) are:

- Any form of crisis information:
  - Suicide hotline
  - Adult protection services
  - Emergency family and single person shelter
  - Homeless shelters and resource centers
  - Domestic Violence shelters
  - Sexual assault hotline
- **FREE** medical
- **FREE** food and location of food banks
- Meals, showers, clothing, and basic needs
- Community legal services
- Provides local telephone numbers nationwide to connect people with human services in their communities
- Services include contact information for food pantries providing **FREE** food
- Also provides help for:
  - Crisis situations
  - Housing and Utilities
  - Health

- Veterans Assistance

- Re-entry to society from rehab or correctional institutions

- More...

• Supported by the United Way and Alliance for Information and Referral Systems (AIRS)

211

This really is the number (like 911) where your local service is available

FoodPantries.org

• A national food pantry website—updated regularly.
Simply **select your state** from the dropdown menu—then find your city.

• A list of all food pantries in your area will appear.

www.foodpantries.org

No phone number listed on website.

Can send an email message (see below)

No email listed. However, you can send a message to them directly from the website by including your name and email address.

County / Local Programs

- Contact your local county office for food programs in your area

- Also check with your local churches, city offices, county offices, and community centers for places offering **FREE** food boxes, **FREE** meals, **FREE** computer training, and more

- The food programs vary from once-a-week service to several times per year—and everything in between—depending on the individual programs

- Some areas even offer **FREE** dinners daily or weekly

Examples:

Macomb County Michigan Food Program

- Provides **FREE** emergency food for those who typically have had a sudden loss of income or other household budget crisis

  o Currently 53 pantries provide food service in Macomb County, Michigan

  o Meals packaged according to need and family size

  o Food package typically lasts five to seven days

(586) 469-6004

Market On The Move

- The 3000 Club, a nonprofit organization, sponsors a program called **Market on the Move**

- Market on the Move rescues and distributes over 30 million pounds of fresh produce every year

- Services the Phoenix and Tucson areas in ARIZONA

- For a $10 donation you may obtain up to 60 pounds of fresh produce

- No income qualifications—open to everyone

- Locations for pickup rotate weekly at various schools, churches, and other locations in the Phoenix and Tucson areas

- Check website and Facebook for dates, times, and locations

the3000club.org

- Find the **Programs** tab at the top of the page (a dropdown menu will appear)

- From the dropdown menu select **Market on the Move**

- The various distribution points, dates, times, and locations will be listed

(623) 374-2559

The 3000 Club
1741 W. Rose Garden, Suites 6 - 9
Phoenix, AZ 85027

facebook.com/the3000club

Check their Facebook page—a list of the produce assortment for the current week is often provided for you to view

FUNERALS

Whether we like it or not, mortality is still at 100%.

Considering average funeral costs range from $7,000 to $10,000, wouldn't it be nice to be able to save anywhere from $3,000 to $5,000 by knowing *one* simple strategy?

Although this may be a delicate subject for many, the fact remains that we *do* have to deal with death at some point.

The most ideal time to deal with this subject is *before* we need to, *before* we lose our loved one(s), and *before* we are unable to think rationally without the debilitating emotions of grief and loss interfering with our judgment.

Burial Benefits for Veterans

Surprisingly, many veterans do not know all or most of the benefits they are entitled to—especially when it comes to their final resting place, and / or basic funeral expenses.

For information on **FREE** Burials for Veterans, please refer to **page 182** of the **VETERAN & MILITARY PROGRAMS** section.

Information on Discounted Caskets

In 1994, the Federal Trade Commission (FTC) made it illegal for funeral homes to force consumers to buy caskets exclusively from the funeral home they are considering working with.

Did you know that funeral homes buy from discount houses like the ones listed below, then increase the prices (sometimes dramatically), and pass those increases on to you?

TIPS:

- A funeral home must accept a casket purchased from a source other than their place of business
- After the funeral director gives a verbal, itemized list of the charges, ask him / her to give you a written itemized bill for everything discussed (this will most likely be done automatically)
- A casket is the largest expense for most funerals

- Purchasing from another source other than the funeral home, will generally save $3,000 to $5,000 on the cost of the casket alone

- You may purchase a casket wholesale, with up to an 80% savings, then have it delivered to the funeral home with no consequence

- A funeral home must provide a written itemized bill, listing all costs of services they will provide

- After you receive a written itemized bill, ask the funeral director to deduct the price of the casket, then purchase your casket wholesale, and have it shipped to the funeral home

- A funeral home cannot insist you purchase a casket from them

If you have further questions, you can always contact the FTC. They will be able to answer any questions you may have.

FTC phone number:

(877) FTC-HELP (877) 382-4357

Cremations

Cremation is another alternative to an underground burial or above-ground vault. Many people are choosing this option for a variety of reasons, including cost.

Requirements vary from state to state, and it is important to check your state for details. For example, some states may require embalming—many do not. Why pay for something that is not required?

It is always important to know your options in order to make an informed decision. Remember whatever you need, may also be purchased at a much lower price from the discount casket companies suggested on the following pages.

Note from Camille:

I know preparing for a funeral can be a very difficult time for most families, and the thought of shopping around and comparing prices may not be an option you have even considered. I also know this can be a time when you may be the most vulnerable, so just contemplate the following: the funeral home would like your business. If they know that you are still looking (which is a good thing to be doing anyway), the initial written quote maybe less. By telling the funeral director that you have not made the final decision to use their facility, there is an extra incentive on their part to make you happy and keep you as a customer.

Furthermore, your loved one may have had some form of insurance to cover a portion (or all) of their final expenses. Do not mention having any form of insurance when you first meet with the funeral director. If they know how much money is available, they may not be as conservative as they could be.

This is why it is so important to consider taking care of business before you need to, and before emotions get in the way of healthy decision-making and judgment. Pre-plan, and consult with an attorney to see if it is in your best interest to pre-pay for any funeral costs.

At the end of this section, there is an opportunity to purchase a phenomenal and comprehensive ebook from the website provided. The author, Susan Noland, addresses just about any conceivable question you may have regarding funerals, including many other cost-cutting funeral options not mentioned in this section. She also provides information on what is required after your loved one is put to rest. The ebook is extremely affordable (less than $10), and will provide links, contact information, and other vital information you may not be aware of. It will also provide contact information for each state, which eliminates the need to search out this information on your own.

Discount Casket Companies

BestPriceCaskets.com

- Has good strategies for how to approach the funeral home
- You may also purchase a casket at this site
- Next-day delivery anywhere in the United States
- This company encourages you to speak with someone from the company before contacting the funeral home
- **FREE** ground shipping

BestPriceCaskets.com

(866) 474-5061
7 a.m. – 11 p.m. daily CST

Universal Casket Company

universalcasket.com

(269) 476-2163
9 a.m. – 5 p.m. EST (Monday – Friday)

Memorials.com

memorials.com

(800) 511-5199

Express Casket

- Same-day or next-day shipping anywhere in the United States
- **Fast delivery** because storage facilities are located around the country
- May view list of showrooms and storage facilities around the country when you select the **ABOUT US** link at the bottom of the page under **Customer Support**
- Located in Texas

expresscasket.com

(888) 448-4001
Open 365-days-a-year (24 / 7)

U.S. Department of Health &Human Services

hhs.gov

(877) 696-6775 (hotline)

Call this number and ask if your state helps with burial costs of any kind

Example:

Michigan ONLY

- Helps with burial costs for those who qualify

- When a person's estate does not have the funds for burial, the SER (State Emergency Relief) assists with burial, cremation, or costs incurred when donating the body to a medical school

- Remains must be in Michigan

Michigan.gov/mdhhs

- Hover over the **Assistance Programs** tab

- From the dropdown menu, select Emergency Relief: Home, Utilities, & Burial

- Then select **Burial**

  - Information on costs for discounted Burial Services will appear

(517) 241-3740

Check with the "Department of Health and Human Services" in your state for similar programs.

OTHER OPTIONS:

Simple Funerals in Michigan (this is the name of the company)

- Funerals from **$975**

- Arrange alternative / nontraditional funeral services

- No fancy limousines, cars, or hearses

- No long visitation service

- No high priced caskets—you can purchase your own

- Simple church service

- Simple graveside service

- Simple burials

- Simple cremation service

- Available in three counties in Michigan:

  - Macomb County

  - Oakland County

  - Wayne County

---

simplefuneralsinmichigan.com

(586) 777-0555 (Macomb County)

(248) 227-1954 (Oakland County)

(313) 382-1181 (Wayne County)

---

*Check to see if your state offers **discounted** funeral services comparable to the above example. Type "**Discounted funeral services (your state)**" in the address bar of your browser.*

WEBSITE FOR MORE INFORMATION TO LOWER FUNERAL COSTS

The website below offers many helpful hints and valuable information for lowering funerals costs in general. Susan Noland compiled an ebook that gives even *more* information on the funeral industry, and all the hidden costs you may be paying because you did not know other options were available.

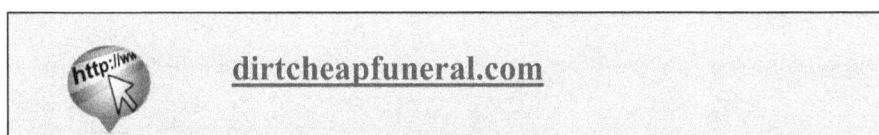

dirtcheapfuneral.com

Survivors' Benefits from Social Security

- A **surviving spouse** may receive a **"Special Lump-Sum Death Payment"** of **$255** if they meet certain requirements

  - Most surviving spouses qualify for this payment

- If there is no surviving spouse, a **surviving child** (or children) may also receive this **Special Lump-Sum Death Payment** of **$255** if they meet certain requirements

- Other Social Security benefits may also be available to the surviving spouse, surviving child (or children), or surviving dependent parent(s), based on specific criteria

  - Those who may be included are the worker's widow / widower / surviving divorced spouse / disabled children / unmarried children under the age of 18 (age 19 if in school) / surviving parent (if dependent on child at the time of his or her death) / mother / father benefits if child under 16 or disabled

- It is best to contact Social Security by telephone for more details regarding qualifications

  - Ask if you qualify for the **"Special Lump-Sum Death Payment"** and **"Social Security Survivors Benefits"**

  - If you quality, they will tell you what documents to bring with you when they schedule your appointment

- You will need to **apply in person** for benefits—no online applications accepted

SocialSecurity.gov or **ssa.gov**

(800) 772-1213 (request appointment)

(800) 325-0778 TTY for deaf or hard of hearing

HOUSING / SHELTER

Miller Trust

A Miller Trust is a special trust that adjusts a person's income downward in an attempt to retain eligibility for certain government benefit programs—generally Medicaid.

It is very important to learn what a Miller Trust offers, as it can make a substantial difference as to whether or not a person qualifies for vitally important government programs.

These trusts can be extremely complex and detailed in nature, and should be drawn up by a seasoned attorney—either one that specializes in estate planning—or an elder law attorney that is familiar with all the specifics a Miller Trust offers.

Important message from Camille:

Senior homelessness is becoming an overwhelming concern in America. Documents like a Miller Trust can often make the difference on whether a senior qualifies for housing or becomes homeless. The consequences are devastating to many seniors across the country, and often go something like this:

- *A senior is on a limited income—often social security.*
- *The annual social security cost of living allowance (COLA) does NOT keep up with inflation.*
- *The landlord raises the rent.*
- *The senior cannot pay the increase with their limited income.*
- *The senior is evicted with no place to go.*
- *The eviction often shows up on a credit report.*
- *Negative credit reporting lowers their credit score.*
- *A low credit score decreases chances to find good housing.*
- *The senior becomes homeless with no mailing address.*
- *The waiting list to obtain subsidized housing is often greater than two years!*
- *Social security does NOT pay social security checks to those without a mailing address.*
- *The senior now is homeless and without any social security income.*
- *The social security check is often the only money they have.*
- *Without an address, they get kicked out of the system.*

- *To get back into the system often takes months after they find housing.*

- *The outcome is often not a positive one.*

- *The undue stress of this cascade of events can cause an elderly person to die prematurely.*

We cannot solve many of the other ongoing issues and situations the elderly encounter, before finding a living space for every senior to call home.

The long-term cost of allowing a senior to continue to live in their own home pales in comparison to putting them in shelters, hotels and motels, nursing homes, and assisted living facilities.

The solutions are many, and one small but important way is to spread the word about this ongoing problem, is to tell everyone you know about a Miller Trust. Those who can and should be providing this information to seniors and concerned parties—simply don't provide it—or don't know this option even exists. This is not a total solution by a long shot. Yet, I know it can often make the difference on whether a person becomes homeless or not.

Other programs are listed in the **HOUSING / SHELTER section**.

Waiver Programs

Waiver programs are another way to help the elderly pay for shelter costs in places like Assisted Living facilities. To qualify for the program, a person needs some help and assistance with several activities of daily living.

Often the person's total monthly income is not enough to pay basic expenses—including the cost of basic shelter. Almost every state has some type of Waiver program that provides financial assistance to help pay the difference between the person's actual income and the shelter / housing cost of the assisted living facility.

Follow the directions on **page 47** of the Waiver section of this resource guide, to find the contact information for your state to see if you qualify for assistance.

HUD Programs

This program allows low-income seniors who are able to live independently on their own—the chance to obtain affordable housing.

The program allows a person to pay only 30% of their gross monthly income for rent and shelter—with 70% of the balance paid by the government.

Remember you must be able to live on your own, and be able to do basic chores like cooking, cleaning, shopping, walking, traveling, grooming, and maintain normal hygiene—in order to qualify for the program.

Your rent increases as your gross income increases—yet it is still extremely helpful to help keep you in your home.

Please contact your **local** Area Agency on Aging (AAA) for more information. (see **page 27** under AAA-Area Agencies on Aging) to see if you qualify.

To contact your *local* Area Agency on Aging

- Go to **ElderCare.acl.gov**
    - Put your **city and state** in the search box
    - A list of **AAA locations** will appear, along with other helpful information

National Council of State Housing Agencies (NCSHA)

These are **STATE-chartered** authorities established to help meet the affordable housing needs of the residents of their states.

National Council of State Housing Agencies:

http://www.ncsha.org/housing-help

- **Select your state** from the map provided
- You will find:
    - The agency name and logo
    - Street address
    - Phone
    - Fax
    - Website
- From the above website, hover over the **About NCSHA** tab at the top of the page.

- Select the **About HFAs** link for more information on the various programs offered.

Contact your **STATE** for various programs and eligibility information, as each state is different.

LICENSE PLATES

Discounted License Plates (also known as "License Tags")

Those with disabilities or handicaps (including seniors), may qualify for **discounted** or **FREE** state license plates(tags). This is different from handicapped plates, as the actual **cost of the plate is discounted**. You will almost **always** have to **ask for this discount** when you renew your license plates, because the information **may not be volunteered**.

TIPS:

- Contact your local Department of Motor Vehicles and ask what is needed to qualify for **"Reduced-Fee License Plates"** (this name may also vary from state to state)

- Call the Secretary of State directly if you are told there is no program available, or if they are not aware of the program(s) in your state—**always ASK** to make sure

- Program **discounts** vary by state, and in some cases may be **FREE**—as with Purple Heart recipients or disabled veterans (you do NOT have to be a veteran to qualify)

EXAMPLE: Michigan ONLY

- In the state of Michigan, a person is entitled to 50% off the price of their annual license tags if they are handicapped, use a wheelchair, and possess a handicapped license plate on their vehicle

  - The vehicle can be a van, mini-van, pickup, passenger vehicle, or motor home that is owned personally, and not by a business or for commercial use

  - The vehicle does not need a wheelchair lift to qualify

- **To apply**: A note from a physician stating use of a wheelchair is submitted—note serves as the application

  - Take the note to the Secretary of State when you renew your tags

- You **may obtain reimbursement** for paying full price for all previous years you met the qualifications

  - You must submit the receipts with your request

Reimbursement Policy

- Find all qualifying receipts from previous years

- Obtain a **Refund Application** in one of two ways:

Dr. Camille S. Superson

1. **Directly from the website**: <u>michigan.gov/sos</u> – From the search box on the website:
   - Type in **Refund Request Form 226**—then select **SOS-Publications & Forms**
   - Scroll down page and select **MI Dept. of State Refund Request Form (A-226)**
   - Fill out form & check the box **Overpayment of Registration Fees** & submit
2. **In person** at the Secretary of State branch office
   - Ask for a "Refund Application"
   - Fill out application and mail with past receipts to the address on the application

Note: If you are the caregiver, and transport your loved one in your own van or mini-van, YOUR vehicle also qualifies. Please note that many vehicles qualify, so please check your vehicle registration to see how the vehicle is classified.

The actual Michigan rule reads as follows:

In the document published by the Secretary of State of Michigan, there is a one-line statement regarding reduced registration fees. Under **"What is the fee for a disability license plate or parking place card"**...please note the following:

"A van owned by a wheelchair user, or by a person who transports a person of his or her household who uses a wheelchair, is eligible for a 50 percent reduction of the standard registration fee for the disabled plate. The van is not required to have wheelchair lift equipment. It can be a full-size window van or a mini-van."

When calling the Secretary of State for clarification, the rule is taken from the Title and Registration Manual on page 42, section C. This rule states that a vehicle must be a **van** or **mini-van** style vehicle to be eligible for the discount.

ANOTHER EXAMPLE FROM THE STATE OF ILLINOIS:

If you qualify (seniors included), there is a flat **$24** fee charged. Details are located in a brochure called **"Reduced-Fee License Plates,"** from the state of Illinois.

> For more information regarding eligibility and qualification, call Illinois Department on Aging:
>
> (800) 252-8966

Personal Note from Camille:

I discovered this 50% discount quite by accident. I had driven my mother's handicapped van to the local Area Agency on Aging, when a total stranger approached me, and said, "Did you know your van qualifies for a 50% discount on the license tags?" I did not.

She proceeded to tell me that she goes out of her way to tell people about this benefit, as most people have no idea they are even entitled to this discount. She further stated that everyone she mentioned this to, was just as surprised as I was!

When the time approached to renew the tags, I mentioned the discount to the lady at the Department of Motor Vehicles service counter. Without flinching, she obliged, and gave the discount.

I asked her why no one ever offered this discount before, knowing that the vehicle qualified for seven years. Her nonchalant reply was, "You never asked!"

How could I have asked for something I didn't know I was entitled to?

*The moral of the story here is to make certain you investigate your state for rules on qualifying for any **discounts** you may be entitled to regarding license tags. You will be amazed at the money you will save!*

Discount License Plates for Purple Heart Recipients

- Nine states offer **FREE** plates and registration
- Eighteen states offer **FREE** plates and have normal registration fees
- The remaining states have a mixture of plate costs and registration fees
- To find out what your state offers:
  - Contact your local **Department of Motor Vehicles** and inquire
  - Check the website for other benefits

www.purpleheart.org

(703) 642-5360, ext. 120 for services

(888) 668-1656 National Headquarters

FREE or Discounted License Plates for Disabled Veterans

If you are a disabled veteran, there is a good chance you qualify for **FREE** or **discounted** license plates. You do not have to be a Purple Heart recipient. It is important to contact the Department of Motor Vehicles for more details, as each state has specific eligibility requirements. Generally, disabilities must be directly related to a service injury, and approved by the Veterans Administration.

- State requirements generally vary from 50% to 100% disability, depending on the state

- Some states issue **FREE** license tags with **FREE** annual renewal

- Some states charge a minimal initial fee with **FREE** annual renewal

- Some states charge an initial fee with minimal or **FREE** annual renewal

- Some states give **FREE** plates to retired veterans

- Some states allow a second plate to be purchased for an additional vehicle

- Some states allow **FREE** travel on specific toll roads for cars displaying a Purple Heart, Legion of Valor, or a Disabled Veteran license plate

*If you are a **VETERAN** or **SENIOR** make sure you **always ask for discounts** wherever you go. This includes grocery stores, restaurants, theaters, theme parks, federal and state parks, airlines, trains, buses, retail stores, telephone companies, and more. Not all give discounts, but many do... and it never hurts to ask. AARP members also receive many discounts with membership.*

*Asking for **discounts** also applies to those with **DISABILITIES** or **SPECIAL NEEDS**!*
*__Always ask for discounts__ wherever you go, including the suggestions listed above. Many places will allow **FREE** admission to the caregiver if they are with someone in a wheelchair. Many theme parks will often move you to the front of the line if you are accompanying someone with a disability or special needs. Always ASK if there are any discounts the business may be offering, because many companies and organizations don't openly advertise their discounts. Asking is the only way you will get them!*

*Check the website: **www.thespeciallife.com/disability-discounts.html** for more suggestions on where to obtain **discounts** for those with disabilities or special needs. Scroll down the page, and select the link on the left that says **Disability Discounts** under the 'Money Matters' area. A list of organizations that offer discounts will appear. This list is not inclusive. This website also offers additional information to questions regarding specific special needs situations.*

MEDICAL ALARMS

Medical alarms are useful and often lifesaving when, and if, a person needs emergency assistance.

Generally, they are used by seniors or disabled persons who live alone. Simply pushing a button on the device (usually worn around the neck or on the wrist like a wristwatch), summons emergency help immediately.

The alarm companies listed below are only a few of the multitude of companies available to you.

The last entry of this section will give quotes to many Top-Rated Medical Alert Companies. You are able to choose more wisely and confidently when determining which company will best suit your needs.

firstSTREET for Boomers and Beyond

- Offers Personal Help Button connected with House Alarm
- A personal notification pendant calls for help for medical or mobile assistance in the home
- Help for:
  - Medical Emergency
  - Accident
  - Fire
  - Burglary
- Offers various options
- 24 / 7 monitoring
- 90-day guarantee
- 100% satisfaction return policy

---

https://www.firststreetonline.com/

This website also offers many different options including supplies, gadgets, clocks, watches, amplified phones, and more...

---

(800) 704-1209

Life Alert

- **FREE** brochure
- Available as a watch or pendant
- Contacts 911 at the push of a button
  - Contacts paramedics
  - Home protection
  - Home invasion
- Monitors:
  - Carbon dioxide gas poisoning
  - Smoke alarms

lifealert.com

Call for price:
(800) 360-0329

Alert-1

- Mobile / Fall Detection units available
- 24 / 7 US-based monitoring
- Same day shipping
- Multi-lingual protection
- Home or on-the-go units
- **FREE** technical support
- 30-day risk-free guarantee
- Landline / Non-Landline units available
- No installation fee
- Monthly fee as low as $24.95
- Order online 24 / 7

www.alert-1.com

(866) 627-7049 (sales)

(866) 957-9837 (orders)
9 a.m. – 6 p.m. EST (Monday – Friday)
10 a.m. – 2 p.m. EST (Saturday)

Top medical alert companies:

Enter the link below into the address bar of your Internet browser.

- Select the **Get Started** button.

- Answer several questions.

- You will be matched with the device(s) that best serve your needs.

- Rate quotes included

- No hidden fees

- No telephone numbers available from the website itself

- Telephone number(s) will be supplied from the individual company once you decide which one to utilize

topmedicalalertcompanies.com

For any concerns or questions, please contact:

admin@topmedicalalertcompanies.com

You will also be able to obtain multiple **FREE** quotes from Top Medical Alarm Companies that are UL-approved monitoring centers.

MEDICAL CLINICS

FREE or **low-cost** medical clinics are generally available in most areas of the country. Links are provided below to help find the clinics closest to you.

**Please check ALL of the websites below, as not all websites have the same information.
This will allow you to compile a more extensive and comprehensive list, so you can add them to the checklist provided at the end of this section.**

Also refer to the **FREE** or **low-cost HEALTHCARE CENTERS** section (**page 54**). The links provided in that section are through the Health Resources & Services Agency (HRSA).

National Association of Free and Charitable Clinics

- This organization provides access to **FREE** or **charitable** clinics in your area

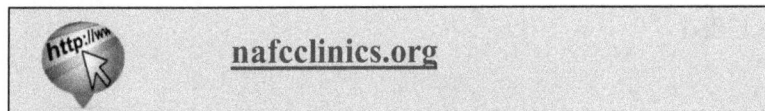

nafcclinics.org

Once you access the website:

- Locate **Find a Clinic** at top of page and select the link
- Enter your **city** and **state** or **zip code** (try both—often brings up additional information)
- List of **FREE** or **charitable clinics** in your area will appear

familywize.org

- Offers many Community Resources, including **FREE** or **low-cost** medical clinics
- This website provides very comprehensive listings of a variety of **FREE** or **low-cost** clinics, including those which are faith based

http://www	**familywize.org**
	(800) 222-2818

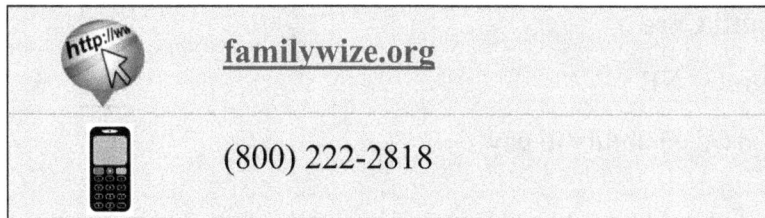

Once you access the website:

- At bottom of page find **Resources** area

- Select the link that says **State Resources**

- Find your state from the dropdown menu and select it

- Various resources including food, shelter, health centers and more, will be provided

- Select the service(s) you may need

- Within your state you will find links for:

  - **FREE** or low-**cost** clinics and services in your area

  - **Food Assistance** for you and your family, including local food banks and pantries—many which are faith based

  - Housing assistance help:
    - Foreclosure
    - Homelessness
    - Subsidized apartments
    - Housing choice vouchers
    - Public housing

  - Utility and weatherization assistance for low income individuals or families

*Check your **LOCAL** area for **FREE** or **low-cost** medical clinics.*
There is often a community center which services your city or township, and they will more than likely have local information readily available to give you.
Also check local hospitals and Catholic charities in your area for more additional information.

EXAMPLES:

1. Choice Family Health Care

- Located in Kearney, NE
- Sliding scale, based on ability to pay

Services offered:

- Breast / cervical cancer screening
- Birth control and pregnancy testing
- HIV testing
- Sexually transmitted infections (STI) testing and treatment

(308) 234-9140

2. Mercy Place Clinic

- Located in Pontiac, Michigan
- Affiliated with St. Joseph Mercy – Oakland Hospital
- Outpatient clinic—cost based on sliding scale
- Provides comprehensive healthcare treatment and prevention to uninsured patients who:
  - Do not qualify under other programs
  - Meet financial guidelines

(248) 333-0840
8 a.m. – 4:30 p.m. EST (Monday – Friday)

3. Aloha Medical Mission

- Located in Honolulu, Hawaii
- **FREE** clinic
- Addresses the needs of an individual whose health is challenged by poverty or poor access to health care

- Provides **FREE** patient surgical care to the indigent
- Only **FREE** full-time dental clinic in Hawaii

(808) 847-3400

4. Primary Care and Hope Clinic

- Located in Smyrna, TN

(615) 893-9390

- Adult medicine / pediatric and women's health services
- Behavioral Health services
- X-ray / Laboratory
- Nutrition
- Sliding fee schedule based on income and family size

NUTRITIONAL SUPPLEMENTS

This section is provided for convenience& informational purposes only.
Consult with your physician or other licensed healthcare professional before taking any
supplements, herbs, or introducing anything new to your daily routine.

Most of the websites below offer nutritional supplements online. Most of them also offer discount pricing and **FREE** shipping with minimum orders.

Total Health Discount Vitamins

- Offers a variety of different companies under one website—all at a discount

- Gluten-free options / Kosher / Health & Beauty / Pet Products

totaldiscountvitamins.com

(800) 283-2833

Swanson Health Products

- Offers massive **discounts**: "Deal of the Day," "Buy One / Get One," and more...

- Vitamins / Herbs / Food Products / Health & Beauty Products / Essential Oils

swansonvitamins.com

(800) 824-4491

Needs.com

- Discounted supplements
- Also offer:
  - Gluten-free options
  - Personal care items
  - Environmental equipment
  - More...
- May request a catalog
- Orders may be placed online

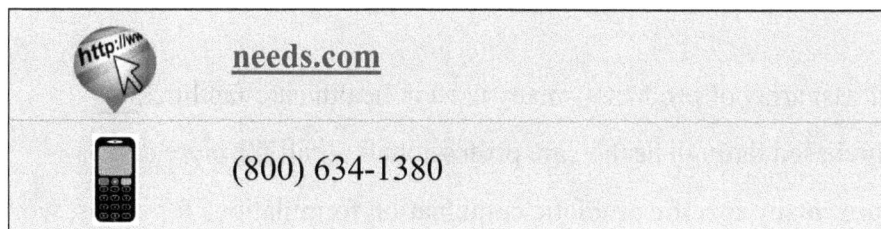

[http icon]	**needs.com**
[phone icon]	(800) 634-1380

Puritan's Pride

- Vitamins / Herbs / Pet Products
- Offer periodic sales: "Buy 1 / Get 2 **FREE**," "Buy 2 / Get 3 **FREE**," and more...
- Gluten-free options
- Health & Beauty / Essential Oils

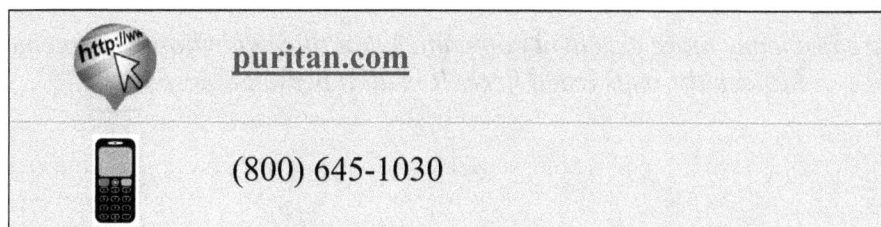

[http icon]	**puritan.com**
[phone icon]	(800) 645-1030

Twin Lab

- Most Twin Lab products are available in capsule, liquid, powder versus tablets, and gel form
- Manufactures and sells other brands like Metabolife, Alvita Teas, as well as REAAL Muscle, Reserveage Nutrition, and NutraScience Labs

http://ww	**twinlab.com**
📱	(800) 645-5626

Metagenics

- Provides a vast array of products—many used in health care facilities
- May be purchased through health care professionals—call for more details
- Manufactures many specific probiotic combination formulations for adults, women, and children
- Many detoxification products also available—please call the company with questions

http://ww	**metagenics.com**
📱	(800) 692-9400

There are many more excellent companies that offer nutritional supplements besides the ones listed here. It is all a personal preference.

PRESCRIPTIONS

The following list of resources will provide either **FREE** or **discounted** prescriptions.

Unless you obtain some or all of your medications **FREE** of charge, the next step involves checking with local pharmacies to see if there are **discounted generics** available for the medications you are taking. Often the cash prices on various generic medications are less expensive than prescription insurance plans or drug cards, especially if they are on the $4 / $10 program listed below. **Discount prescription cards** also provide excellent discounts.

Also refer to: Pharmaceutical Assistance Program and STATE Pharmaceutical Assistance Program (pages 44-45) for FREE medication or help paying medication costs.

A good process to follow:

1. See which medications may be available **FREE** to you (**pages 144 – 145**) from the various resources provided in this guide.

   - The advantage of using this Resource Guide is the ease of finding information quickly. You are able to access any number of medications without having to individually hunt down various manufactures to see if they offer what you need. You are also able to immediately see eligibility requirements and contact information, all in a few easy steps…

2. Check local pharmacies for any **generic medications** you are taking (see **page 147**).

   - Many generics are available: $4 for 30-day supply, $10 for 90-day supply

     o These prices may be less expensive than any insurance or discount card

3. Print out *all* **discount prescription cards** you wish to use (see **pages 145 – 152**) and present them to the pharmacy with any prescription insurance you may have.

   - There is no specific rhyme or reason as to how these discount cards give **discounts**, as you will discover

   - You may have to use different cards for different medications to obtain best possible prices at the exact same pharmacy—can often check the websites to price compare

   - **Discounts** on the *same* discount card for *same* medication may vary from pharmacy to pharmacy *(You may want to re-read this again)*

     o This means that you can use the same discount card, for the same medication, at *different* pharmacies, and prices may vary—can price compare on the websites

   - You *may* be able to use the discount card and your insurance prescription card together for further **discounts**, which may provide even greater savings

This process may involve a little extra time and paperwork in the beginning yet may be well worth the effort, as the dollars you save can add up very quickly!

Many of the discount prescription card websites allow you to check online for the final cost of each medication at *any* of the local pharmacies in your area. Simply enter the information requested. From the comfort of home, you are able to quickly and easily compare prices.

Note from Camille:

You are going to be pleasantly surprised when you discover some of the discount cards also cover PETS! So, everyone in your 'family' is included! ☺

I had completely forgotten about this fact, and it was only while doing some of the final edits of this book, I remembered... and gave it a try.

My Doberman, Grace, took the pain medication Tramadol, and I saved $20.91 per month on her meds!

Take into account that this discount is in 'addition' to the lowest cash price I was already obtaining ($29.25) from one of my local pharmacies. The price decreased to $8.34 using one of the discount cards in this Resource Guide. That savings added up to over $250 per year... and that's for my DOG!

Please also note, the $29.25 price was absolutely the lowest 'cash' price I found. The same medication at different pharmacies was not only higher—it reached upwards toward the $70+ mark at some of the pharmacies consulted. I don't know about you... but to me... it was well worth the effort to take the time to compare prices with the various discount cards. You may be as surprised as I was on how much can be saved on ONE prescription alone!

Free Medication

Pharmaceutical Assistance Program (PAP)

Some drug companies provide assistance on *some* of the drugs they manufacture to people enrolled in Medicare part D, who are experiencing financial hardship, or have no insurance.

medicare.gov/pharmaceutical-assistance-program

- Type **name of drug** in box
- If PAP is available for that drug—drug name appears
  - Click "**Find Drug**"
  - **Name(s) of drug program(s)** (with details) appears AND

- **Pharmaceutical company information** will come up with:
  - o Drug program
  - o Eligibility criteria
  - o Benefits / assistance
  - o Website / contact information

Johnson & Johnson Patient Assistance Foundation

- Helps the uninsured, those whose medications are not covered by insurance, and those who are in financial need, receive **FREE** medications donated by Johnson & Johnson Operating Companies (income requirements vary by medication)

- Forty prescription products available (select **Medications Available** tab at top of page to see if your medication is on the list)

- Select **How to apply** tab (also at top of page) to see if you are eligible for the program

- May apply online if you meet the requirements OR

- **Call the 800 number** and have the application mailed or faxed to you

- You can also view a short **informative video** that explains the program and how to apply—select **About our programs** tab at the top of the page to view

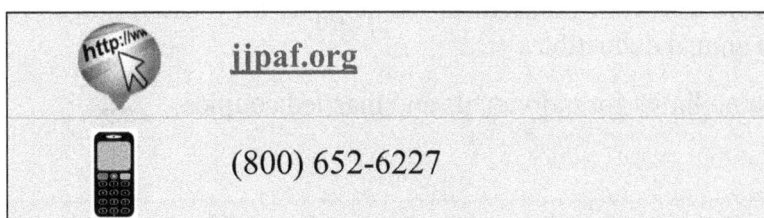

http://	**jjpaf.org**
📱	(800) 652-6227

MedicineAssistanceTool.org

- This website offers various plans for **discounted** or **FREE** medications through various programs

- Simply follow the instructions, and supply them with a list of all your medications

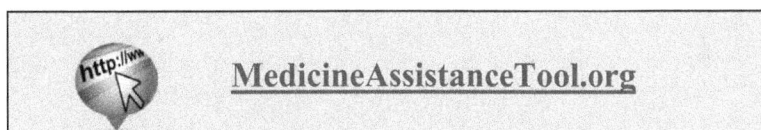

http://	**MedicineAssistanceTool.org**

New York Elderly Pharmaceutical Insurance Coverage (EPIC)

- EPIC is the pharmaceutical assistance program available to New York residents

- Provides financial assistance to seniors 65+ to help with the cost of prescription drugs (generic and name brand)

- Must not be enrolled in Medicaid

- Must be enrolled in or eligible for Medicare Part D prescription plan

- Two tiers available

  - **Fee** or **Deductible Plan**

  - **Based on income** (must be under the limit for both single and married households)

health.ny.gov/health_care/epic
to obtain more information and qualifications for the plan

(800) 332-3742

Extra Help

- Program available to anyone on Medicare to help pay for prescription co-payments, monthly premiums, and annual deductibles

- Must meet income limits for individuals and married couples

socialsecurity.gov/extrahelp

(800) 772-1213

7 a.m. – 7 p.m. (Monday – Friday)

The 3000 Club Medical Reclamation Project

The Medical Reclamation Project saves lives by recovering unused medical supplies, nutritional supplements, educational materials and personal care products and equipment, which are redistributed to people with critical needs on a local, national, and global level.

http://wn	**the3000club.org**
📱	(623) 374-2559 (623) 374-7846 Fax
✉ MAIL	The 3000 Club 1741 W. Rose Garden Lane, Suites 6 – 9 Phoenix, AZ 85027

From the website under the **Our Story** tab, select the link that says **Our Programs** and find **American Medical Aid**. The information describing the program will come right up for you.

Discount Generic Medication

Check with your local pharmacies for best prices on generic medications. Many pharmacies offer a 30-day supply for $4 or a 90-day supply for $10 (or similar programs).

- There are several hundred top generics available
- Not all pharmacies that participate in the $4 / $10 program have the same generics on the list
    - generics on the list may vary from pharmacy to pharmacy
- If one pharmacy does not have your generic medication on their program—check another pharmacy to see if it is on *their* list
- Some pharmacies that participate in this program are:
    - Walmart
    - Costco

- Sam's Club
- Winn-Dixie
- Hy-Vee
- Walgreens
- Publix ($7.50 for a 90-day supply and **FREE** Medication Programs)
- Check other pharmacies as well...

There *may* be an annual fee, depending on the pharmacy.

Always ask if your medication is on the generic list of a participating pharmacy.

Discount Prescription Cards

The price of medications will vary on each discount prescription card.

Different medications will be less expensive with some cards, and other medications will be less expensive with other cards. There is no *best* card for everything. Another thing worth noting is the *same* prescription card for the *same* medication from the *same* pharmacy, may also change occasionally regarding the *cost* of the actual medication (may go up or down in price). This can be a little tricky and confusing, so just be aware that this *does* happen, and don't be surprised if it does. It often works to your advantage when you try another card.

Suggestion: Print out *all* the discount prescription cards you wish to use (the cards are all **FREE** and there is no charge for signing up). Take them to your pharmacy with your prescriptions. Use the cards that give the best **discounts** on the medications you are taking.

Many of the websites will allow you to check the price of your medication online, as well as provide a list of the local pharmacies in your area. That way, you will know the price of your medication at *each* pharmacy location before you actually fill the prescription. These prices may vary from pharmacy to pharmacy—and also by medication—using the exact same card.

The Discount Prescription Cards may sometimes be used in conjunction with an insurance prescription card, and you *may* be entitled to further **discounts**.

These discount prescription cards are able to save families hundreds (if not thousands) of dollars annually, depending on the amount of medication used in the household.

1020 Rx Health Benefit Plans

- Drug **discounts** of $10 / $20 / $40 prescriptions based on tier chosen
- Must pay a monthly fee based on coverage you choose
- Actual drug cost can be calculated on website

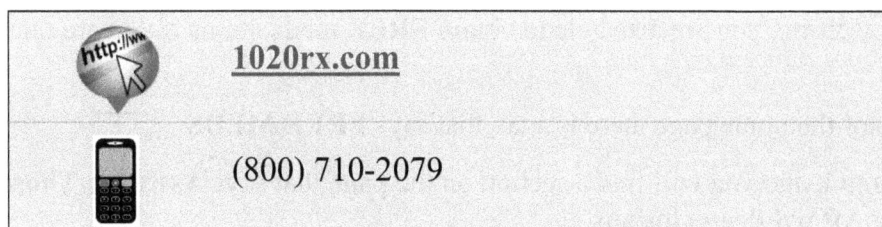

http://	**1020rx.com**
📱	(800) 710-2079

LARx Prescription Savings Program

- For residents of Los Angeles, California ONLY
- **FREE** card obtained from website
- Save 5% to 65% on brand and generic drugs
- Use at all participating pharmacies in Los Angeles County
- Price compare on website from various local pharmacies

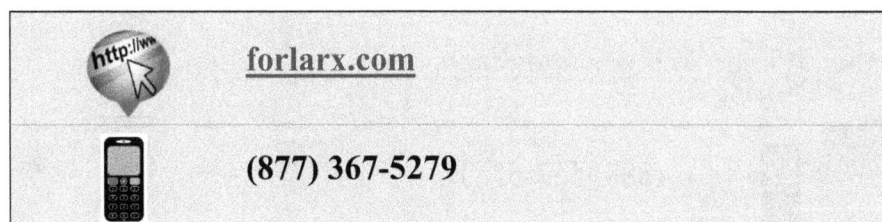

http://	**forlarx.com**
📱	**(877) 367-5279**

Your Rx Card

- Fill out the form
- Print off card from website and take to pharmacy
- Up to 75% off FDA approved drugs

yourrxcard.com

(866) 561-1926
9 a.m. – 3 p.m. CST (Monday – Friday)

- From this website, you are also able to obtain **FREE** medications if you are unable to afford them

- At the top of the home page there is a tab that says **FREE MEDS**

- Select this link and you will find a section on the page that says **Assisting Those Who Are Unable to Afford Prescriptions**

- Select the link that says Patient Assistance Programs

- Follow the directions to also obtain **FREE** coupons directly from the manufacturer on many medications

- There are also many other options available

Medication Card

- Print off card from website and take to pharmacy

medicationcard.net

(888) 553-5751

Simple Savings Card

- Can save up to 80% on prescriptions
- Print off card from website and take to your pharmacy

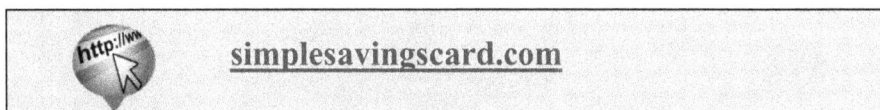

simplesavingscard.com

Easy Drug Card

- Save up to 75% on prescriptions
- Print off card from the website and take to pharmacy
- Pet medications also covered (only those that are also used for humans)
- Able to check online for drug prices at local pharmacies

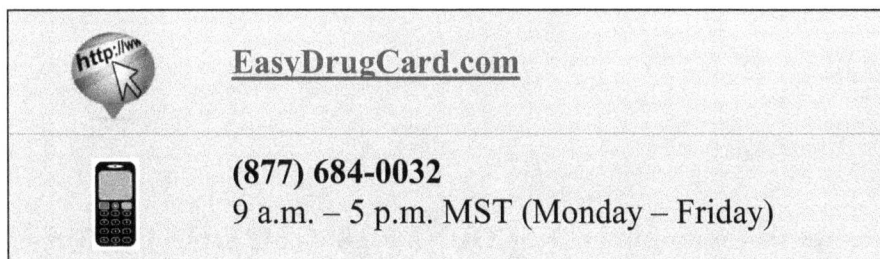

EasyDrugCard.com

(877) 684-0032
9 a.m. – 5 p.m. MST (Monday – Friday)

GoodRx.com

- Type the **name of the drug** in the search area that says **Find the Lowest Price**
- A list prices from various pharmacies in your area will come up

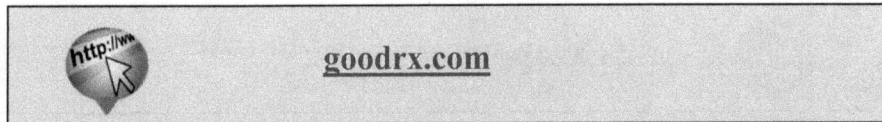

goodrx.com

Other Discount Prescription Cards are included in the links below

The websites below all require printing the card from their website, and submitting the card to the pharmacy with your prescription.

This is by no means an inclusive list, as there are more and more Discount Prescription Cards available as time goes by.

npsncard.com

honestdiscounts.com

pscard.com

rxassist.org

The websites that follow offer DISCOUNT PRESCRIPTION CARDS as well as *other* valuable resources and information.

- Many of the additional resources are **FREE**—please review to see which resources may be able to assist you, besides the **discounts** offered on prescription medications
- Available to everyone (as many of the resources are)—some even include PETS!
- The following websites are included in this section for your convenience, because they offer other services in addition to their prescription discount cards

Familywize.org

This website also offers many Community Resources, including **FREE** or **low-cost** medical clinics, as well as **discounts** on **pet** medications.

familywize.org

(800) 222-2818

- At the top of the page type in the **drug you are looking for** and **your zip code** in the search boxes provided—best price quotes from local pharmacies will appear

- At the bottom of the page, find the **Resources** area and select **State Resources**

- **Enter your state** in the search box provided

- Select any of the resources you may need help with

You will find links for:

- **FREE** or **low-cost** clinics and services in your area

- **Food assistance** for you and your family, including local food banks and pantries

- Housing assistance help:
  - Foreclosure
  - Homelessness
  - Subsidized apartments
  - Housing choice vouchers
  - Public housing

- **Utility and weatherization assistance** for low income individuals or families

RxSavingsPlus.com

- Besides **discounts** on your prescriptions, this card also gives discounts on **pet** medications (only those that are also used for humans)
  - Please also check the $4 / $10 programs available (as described previously) if your pet is also on generic medication
- 10% discount on Minute Clinic health service or screening, up to $10 per person per visit

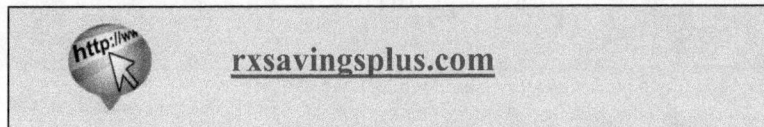

rxsavingsplus.com

Nacorx.org

- Besides discount prescription coverage, website provides information on:
  - Health topics
  - Food and nutrition
  - Recipes
  - Physical fitness
  - Men's and women's health issues
  - Natural and Alternative Treatments
- **Pet** medications are also covered (only those that are also used for humans)
  - Please also check the $4 / $10 programs available (as described previously) if pet is also on generic medication

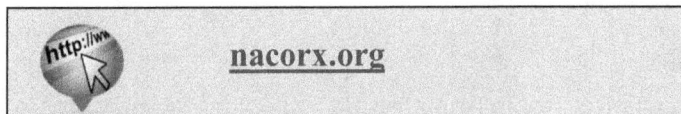

nacorx.org

Coast2CoastRx.com

- This card also provides **discounts** for:

  - Dental

  - Vision

  - Laboratory and Imaging

  - Veterinary services

  - Diabetic supplies and equipment

  - Prescriptions (for both humans and **pets**)

    o Pets must be taking the same medications humans take

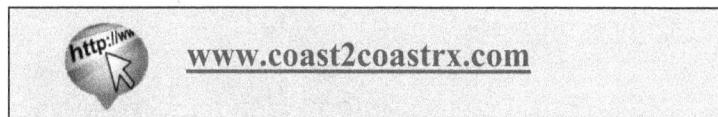

www.coast2coastrx.com

There is a tab to the right of the page that says **Print Your FREE Card for Residents of Townships, Cities, or Counties.** Select the link, then select your **City, County or Township.** Not all participate. Those that do are highlighted when you select the tab and identify your local city, township, or county. The website says you may use cards anywhere in the United States, even if your city, township, or county is not listed. Select **Prescription Card** tab at the top.

Also, select the tab at the top of page for **More Benefits**. Details are provided for each benefit.

RESPITE CARE

Area Agency on Aging

Each local community has its own Area Agency on Aging (AAA). Please refer to the **GOVERNMENT AGENCY RESOURCES** section (**page 26**) to find your local AAA chapter. Call and ask your local Area Agency on Aging if they have an "**Out-of-Home Respite Care**" program. If they do, and depending on the state—the cost may be a total out-of-pocket expense, or there may be a sliding scale option. There are also other Respite programs and services available for caregivers through your local AAA for **FREE**. Always check your **local** AAA for more information.

Website again for
National Area Agency on Aging:

n4a.org

Local contact information may be obtained from the above website.

Out-of-Home Respite Care

- Out-of-Home Respite provides care to a qualified recipient outside the home

- Families or individuals are free to relax, recharge, or simply enjoy the time in their own home or surroundings for a designated period of time

- Government programs may change from time to time, so always ask the person you are speaking with, if there are similar programs available in your state, county, or region

Again, remember that qualifications, eligibility, and fees may vary regarding Out-of-Home Respite Care—depending on the state, county, or region. Fees generally range from a sliding scale, all the way up to a total out-of-pocket expense for this service.

*Contact your **LOCAL** Area Agency on Aging for similar programs.*
Remember, the names of the programs may also vary slightly depending on where you live.

Easter Seals

- Easter Seals assists those with **special needs** or **disabilities** including: **children**, **young adults**, **adults**, **seniors**, and **veterans**, by providing medical and social services

- **Services:**

  - Medical rehabilitation

  - Respite care

  - Transportation solutions for caregivers & more…

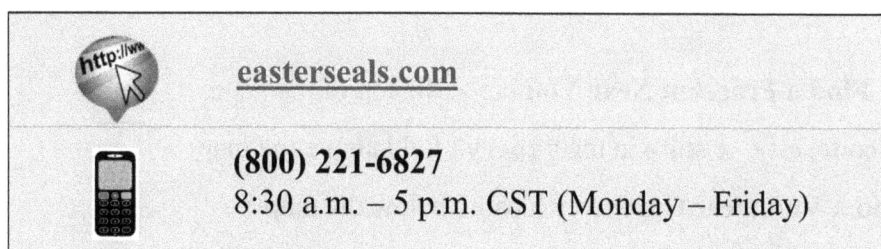

easterseals.com

(800) 221-6827
8:30 a.m. – 5 p.m. CST (Monday – Friday)

- At the top of the page select tab that says **What We Do**

- You will see links for Senior, Adults, Children, Autism, and Veteran Services

- Select the link that applies to your specific need

National Volunteer Caregiving Network

- The primary goal of this program is to provide assistance to homebound neighbors with chronic health conditions or disabilities—creating independent living through various volunteer programs

- Available in many areas of the country, but not all

- Provides assistance in the following non-medical areas:

  - Shopping / errands

  - Reading

  - Bill payment

  - Minor home repairs / yard work

  - Light housework

  - Transportation to medical and other appointments

- Respite care for family caregivers
- Visiting

nvcnetwork.org

May send questions via email by selecting the **Contact** Us tab at the top of page

(512) 582-2197

- Select the **Find a Program Near You** tab at the top of the page.
- Enter **zip code, city,** or **state** in the **"query"** field above the map.
- Select **Find a Volunteer Caregiver** located below the map.
- Fill out the requested information.
- Click the **Send Request** button and someone will contact you within three business days.

Please feel free to also call the number above if you need further assistance. They will be more than happy to assist you.

ARCH National Respite Locator

archrespite.org

(703) 256-2084

- Website allows you to search for **local** respite programs in your state
- On left side of the home page hover over **Respite Locator**
  - Then select **Respite Funding and Caregiver Supports**
  - **Select your state** from the map provided for detailed local **respite** choices and various funding to help pay for care

United Way

- Check your local United Way chapter to find all the services they offer, including:

  - Helping the homeless

  - Respite care for caregivers and housekeeping services

  - May offer **money** for respite care in your area, depending on where you live

    - Talk directly to the staff to receive funds

  - **FREE** or **reduced** dental programs may be available

http://	**unitedway.org**
	(703) 836-7112

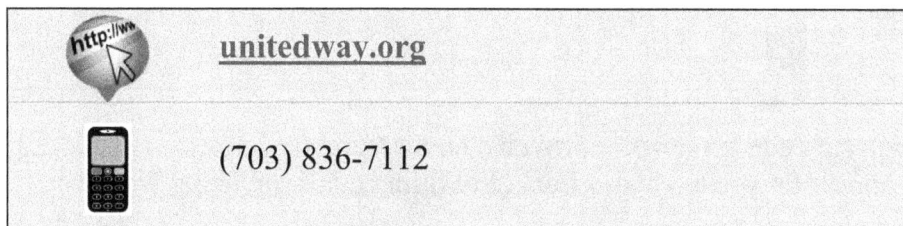

- Select the link in the upper right-hand corner **Find Your United Way**

- Enter **zip code** then select **SUBMIT**

- Call the number provided for your location and ask what programs they offer

Please refer to:
MISCELLANEOUS ORGANIZATION section (page 190) and scan through the
list of organizations for additional 'respite care' resources

Paid Respite Care

At some point, it may be necessary to contact an agency and hire a paid caregiver.

There are a variety of reasons you may need to do this, as dynamics are constantly changing within families.

Although you may never need this service, is important to prepare for this possibility and begin to search for an agency which can potentially assist you, should you need them in the future.

Another alternative would be to hire a *private* caregiver:

You are able to obtain quality help for less than you would pay an agency, and the caregiver is able to make a little more. There is no middleman involved.

This is often a win-win situation, as it allows both parties to negotiate fees directly with one another and discuss more openly what is expected from each party.

One place to obtain private caregivers is through Carelinx, a professional caregiver marketplace. Caregivers are already pre-screened with full background checks, and are bonded and insured before you hire them. There is a 15% service fee for each invoice, which covers the benefits Carelinx provides. Contact Carelinx directly for more information.

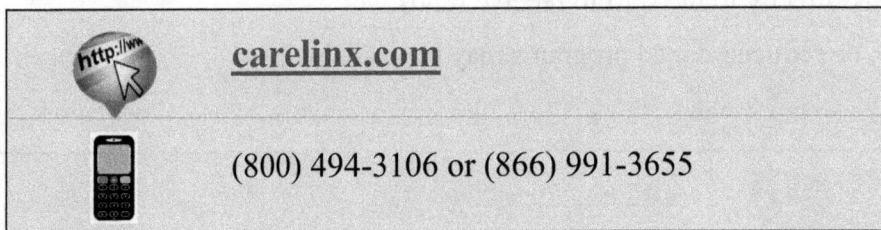

carelinx.com

(800) 494-3106 or (866) 991-3655

- **Enter your zip code** in the space provided on the Carelinx website—a list of caregivers in your area will appear for you to choose from after filling out form listing your specific needs

If hiring through an agency, you may want to ask the following questions:

- Do they charge reasonable rates for services provided?

- Are there any additional hidden costs you may not be aware of?

- Are there **discounts** available if you need a live-in caregiver, or if you need someone on an ongoing basis every week, or month?

- Are the caregivers carefully scrutinized & trained before they ever go out on assignment?

- Do you resonate with the caregiver assigned to your loved one?

    - If not, will they carefully provide someone else who may be more compatible with you and / or your loved one?

- Are all your questions answered to your satisfaction?

Preparing yourself 'before' you need help will save a lot of time later, when you actually do need this service.

THERAPY ANIMALS/ SERVICE ANIMALS

Therapy animals are used for comfort in institutional settings like hospitals and nursing homes, hospice, schools, disaster areas, in a person's home setting, or to help those with learning disabilities.

- Dogs, cats, horses, donkeys, pigs and a variety of other animals have been used, depending on the situation

- Therapy animals are privately owned, and generally return home with the owner at the end of the visit

Service animals (which are primarily dogs), help disabled individuals by performing tasks that aid and assist the disabled person throughout the day.

- The disabilities vary by individual need—so do the tasks the service animals perform

- Service animals are protected by federal law under the Americans with Disabilities Act (ADA)

- There are many disabilities that quality—both physically and mentally—the list is extensive (see website link on next page)

- Service dogs are often identified by wearing a vest or tag, which easily lets the public know they are service dogs

- Service animals are almost always **FREE**—you simply need to apply for them

  - There may be a waiting list of two years or more—it helps to apply as soon as possible

  - You can always cancel if the animal is not needed

Emotional support dogs provide comfort and support to those suffering from various emotional and mental conditions, including autism.

These dogs are also protected by federal law under the Americans with Disabilities Act (ADA).

- Emotional support dogs are often identified by wearing a vest or tag, which lets the public know they are emotional support dogs

- The Fair Housing Amendments Act (FCAA) protects individuals by allowing their emotional support dogs to be able to live with them regardless of pet policies that do not allow animals

- The website below will also provide a list of emotional disabilities that qualify for dogs

officialservicedogregistry.com

- This website provides details on registering a service, therapy, or emotional support dog

- This website also provides information on other questions you may have, including a **list of disabilities (both physical and emotional) that qualify for these dogs**

  - Select the links that say **Service Dog Information—Emotional Dog Information—**and **Therapy Dog Information—**for **more details—**including the list of disabilities that qualify under each category

The websites below provide locations and contact information to obtain these animals.

Canine Companions for Independence

- Dogs and follow up are provided **FREE**

- Provide:

  - Service dogs

  - Skilled companion dogs

  - Facility dogs

  - Hearing dogs

  - Assistance dogs for veterans

cci.org

(800) 572-BARK (2275)

PAWS With A Cause

- Provide:
  - Service dogs
  - Hearing dogs
  - Assistance dogs
  - Seizure response dogs
  - Service dogs for children with Autism
- Dogs are **FREE** to those who qualify—available in approximately 30 states
  - Qualifications vary depending on the type of dog required
- Select **CLIENT APPLICATION** tab at the top of the page and fill out the form—application requests are available only certain times of each year, with a $25 fee. Always inquire for times.
- Application enrollment period for 2021: January 4, 2021 through March 31, 2021.

	pawswithacause.org For those children younger than the PAWS minimum age requirement, please visit the website: **www.assistancedogsinternational.org** for possible assistance in finding programs for these children
	(616) 877-7297 (National Headquarters: Wayland MI) 8 a.m. – 4:30 p.m. EST (Monday – Friday) **(248) 619- 9201** (SE Michigan Regional Office-Troy, MI). Hours by appointment
	Email: **paws@pawswithacause.org** (for both locations)
	National Headquarters: 4646 South Division Wayland, MI 49248

Guardian Angels Medical Service Dogs

- Located primarily in Florida, with divisions in Michigan and Illinois

- Dogs are **FREE** to qualified recipients / $50 application fee

- In-depth application process allowing customized training to meet recipients' personal challenges and needs

  - Once approved—placed on waiting list

- Wait time: one to two years for Post-Traumatic Distress Disorder (PTSD) dog—three to four years (can be up to 10 years) for other disabilities

- Two other options available to speed the waiting time:

  - **Foster Pairing / Foster Training**

    o Take dog home within first month

    o Basic training and manners generally already done

    o Must commit to classes once a week

      - Offered on Thursdays and Saturdays—may attend both

    o Must pay all upkeep, food, spaying or neutering (one time charge)

    o Must pass final test with chosen dog to make sure dog and owner work well together

    o Once officially paired, will receive vest and ID cards

  - **P.E.T.S. (Pets Evaluated and Trained for Service) Program**

    o You already have your own dog—confirmation of disability to have a service dog is required.

    o If they believe your dog has what it takes to be transformed into a service dog, they will train both you and your dog for a minimum of six months to be able to work together effectively.

    o You must be physically and cognitively able to attend classes with your dog.

    o Pricing depends on amount of training involved.

    o Contact any of the numbers on the next page, and ask for more information.

www.medicalservicedogs.org

(800) 398-6102 (general information)
Option 1: General information
Option 2: Recipients and applications
Option 3: Donor relations
Option 4: Fostering and training questions

Florida numbers:

(352) 425-1981 (Central Florida)
(813) 294-9611 (Tampa Area)
(239) 877-3012 (Naples – S. Florida)
(301) 806-6953 (Panhandle)

(815) 762-0563 (Illinois Division)

(248) 904-0579 (Michigan Division)

(412) 298-9940 (Pittsburgh Division)

(239) 300-5248 (Fostering & Training Q's)

Select the **CONTACT US** tab at the top of the page to send email directly

Leader Dogs for the Blind

- Provides **FREE** leader dogs for the blind

For full details, see **page 98**.

Service Dog Central

- Offers information on many topics regarding service dogs, disabilities, laws, and more...

  - Besides looking for service dogs, you may want to browse this entire site later, as there is a lot of useful information on the site which may be helpful to you

servicedogcentral.org

Unfortunately, no phone number
or email address is available

- To obtain a service dog:

  - On the left side of the page, under 'Frequently Asked Questions' select **How do I find a service dog?**

  - Once you select this link, find the list of **green links** located in the center of the page. The links most relevant in finding a service dog for you are:

    - **American Dog Trainers Network**: List of organizations (by state) that provide both *service* and *assistance* dogs, including:

      - Hearing Dogs

      - Guide Dogs

      - Search and Rescue Dogs

      - Support Dogs

      You will need to call each contact directly to find the specific *types* of dogs they offer.

    - **Wolfpacks**: List of organizations (by state) that *provide* service dogs, as well as those that *train* service dogs, including facility, hearing, and skilled companion dogs

      - Once you **select your state**, many of the contacts will also specify what *type(s)* of service dogs they provide

TRANSPORTATION FOR SENIORS AND THE DISABLED

Obtaining adequate transportation for seniors and disabled Americans is a serious ongoing nationwide problem. Many of these individuals do not own an automobile, or have family members or friends to drive them to places like grocery stores, doctor visits, and other places of interest. Some of these individuals are disabled—some are not—and not being able to have the freedom to travel to various destinations can lower their moral and the ability to be self-sufficient.

Besides finding viable **FREE** or **low-cost** public transportation, it is also important to also contact the Area Agency on Aging in your area, as well as your city's senior centers and community centers for more information regarding door-to-door transport services in your area.

These services are generally limited to seniors (over the age of 60 – 65), and those with disabilities.

In the address bar of your browser, type in:

"(Your city and state) community centers"
"Community centers (your city and state)"

"(Your city and state) senior centers"
"Senior centers (your city and state)"

"Area Agency on Aging (your state)"

Examples:
"Detroit Michigan community centers"
"Community centers Los Angeles, CA"

"Buffalo New York senior centers"
"Senior Centers Denver, CO"

"Area Agency on Aging Houston, TX"

To find these additional transportation services, call the community centers and senior centers in your city for door-to-door transportation services for seniors and those with disabilities.

Cost:

- Varies from service to service

- Generally partial voucher plus percentage and / or cost per mile (varies)

OR

- Flat rate minimum mileage plus additional charge per mile

Examples:

In Scottsdale, AZ… there are three options to choose from.

Cab Connection:

- For Scottsdale residents only
- Provides door-to-door rides for seniors over the age of 65
- 20 vouchers given per month—each voucher good for (1) one-way trip, or 10 round trips per month
- Customer pays 20% of fare—each voucher worth maximum of $10
- Over $10 voucher maximum—customer pays difference
- Wheelchair accessible
  - Call 24 hours ahead for wheelchair transport

📱	Contact Cab Connection for information packet **(480) 312-7696**
MAIL	7447 East Indian School Rd., Suite 205 Scottsdale, AZ 85251

Valley Metro RideChoice

- For Scottsdale residents only
- Residents must be American Disabilities Act (ADA) paratransit certified
- Utilizes Lyft, taxis, and wheelchair-accessible vehicles to transport passengers
- Cost per ride:
  - Up to 8 miles - $3
  - Additional miles - $2 per mile

Dial-A-Ride (Valley Metro Regional & East Valley Dial-A-Ride)

- Is an origin-to-destination advanced reservation transportation service for seniors and persons with disabilities
- Services seniors age 65 and older, and those with disabilities

- Scottsdale **Dial-A-Ride** services Scottsdale, Chandler, Mesa, Gilbert, Tempe, Paradise Valley
- Services ADA and non-ADA trips
- Wheelchair access
- Cost:
  - ADA - $4
  - Non-ADA - $4 for first 5 miles + 50cents per mile (6 – 15 miles) + $1 per mile over 16 miles

For more information: **(480) 633-0101**

Other Dial-A-Ride services available in most cities across the nation.

Dial-A-Ride

This is a national origin-to-destination advanced reservation transportation service for **seniors and persons with disabilities, and those who can't use standard fixed route transit systems** to travel to medical appointments, employment, school, and grocery stores.

- Available in most states

- Transports seniors (over age 65) and those with disabilities who are unable to use normal public transportation and routes

- Each state has own criteria to use the service

- 24 hour advance notice is generally required

- Price varies from state to state

  - Very low fares—generally with minimum and maximum costs per trip

    - Generally $3 - $3.50 to board

    - Maximum trip generally from $9 -$10.50 per trip

    - Can be as low as $2 each way (rarely) - depends on city

- Wheelchair accessible

- No general / national website and phone number available

- Contact your city for more details

- In the search box of your browser type in "**Dial-a-ride (city and state)**"

  - **Examples:**

    - **"Dial-A-Ride Denver, Colorado"**

    - **"Dial-A-Ride Seattle, Washingtom"**

- Call the phone number to schedule a ride (make sure you allow 24 hour advanced notice)

- When in doubt, contact your local Area Agency on Aging to assist you

Wheelchair Getaways

- Nationwide network

- Specializes in short and long-term accessible van rentals

- Deliver fully-equipped vans to:

  - Your home

  - Your business

  - Airport arrivals

  - Other destinations

- Provides:

  - **FREE** information on accessible accommodations and attractions

  - 24-hour emergency assistance

  - An opportunity to rent a van before purchasing one

accessiblevans.com

- Enter **zip**, **city** or **airport** in the **Find A Location** box

  - Local contact information (including phone number) will appear

(888) 432-8790 or (877) 275-4915

- Check website for more information.

- Renting may be a more cost-effective alternative rather than purchasing a fully equipped van outright, especially if not needed on a daily basis.

This is a viable alternative to the huge investment of purchasing a personal motorized van, especially if transport of the handicapped individual is minimal.

Please refer to:
MISCELLANEOUS ORGANIZATIONS (page190)

Read through the list to find the organizations that offer 'transportation' services.

Please refer to:
ADDITIONAL TRANSPORTATION HELP (page 175)
and:
Your local AREA AGENCY ON AGING (page 26)—ask for 'transportation services'

Program of All-Inclusive Care for the Elderly (PACE)

Program of All-Inclusive Care for the Elderly (PACE) uses a combination of Medicare and Medicaid benefits for some or all of the long-term care needed. This program allows people to live in their home instead of going into a nursing home. A monthly fee could be charged.

Qualifications:

- Eligible for Medicare / Medicaid benefits
- Age 55+
- Live in PACE area
- Eligible for nursing home care

Exclusions:

- CANNOT be enrolled in the Waiver Program at the same time
- NOT available in every state

http://w	**npaonline.org** (National Pace Association)
📱	(703) 535-1565

- Select the box that says **Find a PACE Program**
- Type in your **zip code** or **select your state** from the map
- It will bring up all the contact information if your State has as PACE Program

FREE Transportation

These are generally **COUNTY** and **CITY** programs.

Many counties and municipalities have services to provide **FREE** and / or affordable transportation to **seniors** and / or **physically disabled adults**.

Besides the local government resources provided in this guide, check your county and city for additional local resources, including churches and local volunteer organizations or schools.

There are also many local alternatives, including shuttle services and other public transportation services that are available **FREE** or **low-cost** to seniors and those with disabilities.

In the address bar in your browser type in:

"FREE transportation services for seniors (your city and state)"

Example:

- "FREE transportation services for seniors Los Angeles, CA"

This should bring up a variety of **FREE** or **low-cost** transportation services in your local area.

Please refer to:

MISCELLANEOUS ORGANIZATIONS section (page 190) and scan through the list for the organizations that offer 'transportation' services, including volunteer organizations

Also refer to:

Angel Wings For Veterans FREE airline transport for the veteran and their caregiver see (page 176).

And:

Your local AREA AGENCY on AGING (page 26)—ask what 'transportation' services may be available to you FREE or low-cost

EXAMPLE: Macomb County, Michigan

This service is **FREE** to those who qualify.

Eligibility

- Must be a Macomb County, Michigan resident

- Have a documented need for medical treatments

- Do not have access to public transportation

- Do not live with someone who owns and drives a vehicle

- Caregiver must assist any rider who is unable to meet the vehicle curbside without assistance, and must provide the name of the person who will help the rider board and depart the vehicle if assistance is necessary

- Rides must be scheduled at least one week in advance, two weeks is preferred

- Must provide 24-hour notice of ride cancellation

- Must specify special needs, such as a hydraulic wheelchair lift

Macomb County, Michigan:
mca.macombgov.org/MCA-Home

(586) 469-5225

- From the website type in **Transportation Services** in the search box

- Select MCA-Transportation

  - **List of Program Guidelines** and additional information will appear

- Requests for transportation made during regular business hours:
  8:30 a.m. – 5 p.m. EST (Monday – Friday)

- Transportation operates between the hours of 6 a.m. & 4:30 p.m. (EST) departing for the final destination by 2 p.m.

Contact your **COUNTY or CITY / TOWN / VILLAGE** for program and eligibility information.

Additional Transportation Help

Independent Transportation Network (ITN) is an organization that provides dignified transportation and lifelong mobility for seniors in certain areas of the country, with additional services being added on a regular basis.

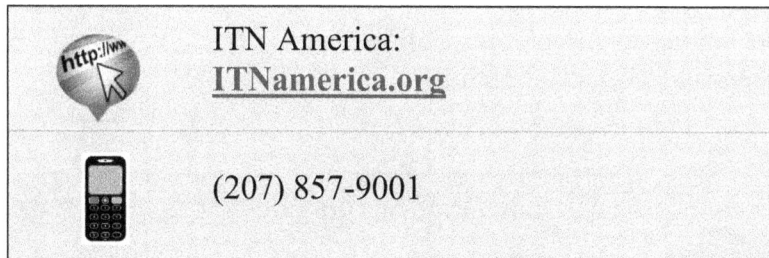

ITN America:
ITNamerica.org

(207) 857-9001

- Select the link that says **Find Your ITN** in the upper right-hand side of the site

- Map of United States will appear

- **Find your area on the map** (if it is listed) and select the markers for local contact information

- Older adults who join become dues-paying members and pre-fund a transportation account

  - Must be 60 years old or visually impaired to join

  - Tipping NOT expected or permitted

  - Available 24 / 7

Discounts are available for advanced notice or for shared rides.

Note: *Only select parts of the country are served.*

VETERAN & MILITARY PROGRAMS

In addition to all the resources outlined in this book, veterans may qualify for additional resources, including the resources listed below. Please also note that some of the programs include the **caregiver** or **spouse of a veteran**.

Caregivers of veterans, through the Department of Veterans Affairs (VA), may receive up to 30 days of respite care per year (depending on the program).

> VA Caregiver Support Line:
>
> **(855) 260-3274**
> 8 a.m. – 8 p.m. EST (Monday – Friday)

You may be surprised at all the benefits you may qualify for and are entitled to, including a monthly stipend, and depending on the program.

Program of Comprehensive Assistance for Family Caregivers

Veterans may appoint one primary (main) caregiver and two secondary caregivers (who serve as backup to primary caregiver).

Beginning January 1, 2020: Designated primary family caregivers of eligible veterans are granted privileges to commissaries, post exchanges, and recreational facilities if recognized under the program.

Angel Wings for Veterans (AWV)

AWV's mission is to ensure that no financially stressed wounded warrior, veteran, or adversely affected family member is denied access to distant specialized medical evaluation, diagnosis, counseling, treatment, or rehabilitation for a lack of means of long-distance medical air transportation, or shorter distance ground travel. WV also provides travel assistance related to acquiring a Service Dog, or other programs. Contact AWV for more details.

http://	angelwingsforveterans.org
📱	(757) 318-9174 (757) 464-1284 Fax
@	info@angelwingsforveterans.org May also email directly from the website: Select the **Contact** tab at the top of the home page and fill out information as requested.
MAIL	4620 Haygood Rd. Suite 3 Virginia Beach, VA 23455

- For details on the program select **ABOUT US** at the top of the page for information on both air and ground transportation
- To seek assistance select **REQUEST ASSISTANCE** at the top of the page
  - Select **Commercial Airline Assistance OR Request Ground Transportation**
  - Fill out the form and submit (fastest way), OR call the number above

Attorneys

- Online military lawyers
- You ask questions and receive answers

http://	justanswer.com/Military-law

Lawyers Serving Warriors®

Lawyers Serving Warriors is part of the National Veterans Legal Services Program (NVLSP), a nonprofit organization. Their mission is to ensure veterans and active-duty personnel obtain all benefits they are entitled to from the government.

- The NVLSP is an *extremely* important resource for Veterans

- Take the time to check all the services offered on the website

- Remember, if you are a veteran or active duty personnel and you have been denied the benefits you are entitled to, please contact NVLSP, and they will help you

- This service is **FREE** to all veterans from all eras **with disability issues**, who are experiencing difficulties obtaining the benefits they are entitled to

- Representation includes:

  - Disability

  - Discharge

  - Veteran benefits

---

nvlsp.org

- At the top of the Home page find the tab **What We Do**

- Dropdown menu will appear

- Select Class Actions

- View cases where veterans and *spouses* were wrongfully denied benefits they were entitled to (over $3 billion recovered)

(202) 265-8305, ext. 152

info@nvlsp.org

Canine Companions for Independence

- Dogs and follow up are provided **FREE**

- Provide:

    - Service dogs

    - Skilled companion dogs

    - Facility dogs

    - Hearing dogs

    - Assistance dogs for veterans

http://	**cci.org**
📱	(800) 572-BARK (2275)

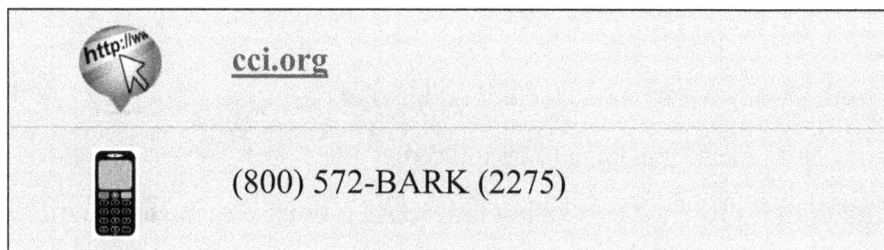

Please refer to:

THERAPY ANIMALS / SERVICE ANIMALS section (page 161)

*This section provides many important links/websites to assist you or your loved one
in obtaining a service dog/emotional support dog, if you are physically or emotionally disabled.*

Department of Veterans Affairs (VA)

This is a *federal* agency that should be able to handle most of the military claims, benefits, and other programs and services veterans qualify for. In many cases, there have been massive delays processing claims, so it is important to be persistent and follow up frequently to check the status of each and every claim filed. This agency should also be able to answer all questions related to veterans and their families.

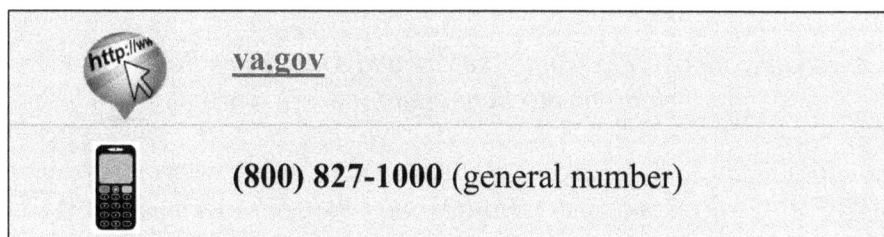

http://	**va.gov**
📱	**(800) 827-1000** (general number)

Aid and Attendance Benefit

This benefit is an Enhanced Pension offered through the Veterans Administration, and is a pension benefit most people are not aware of. It also includes the **surviving spouse.** This benefit **will help pay some of the long-term costs** of In-Home Care, Board and Care, Assisted Living, and Nursing Home Care to any veteran who has served at least one day during wartime before the Gulf War. The amount allowed will vary from **$1,244** for a widow to **$3,032** for two veterans per month, and is **tax-free.** This benefit is provided *in addition* to basic pension benefits or disability compensation.

To qualify:

- Age 65 or older

- Must meet income and net worth requirement (house and car are exempt)

- Must need assistance for two or more activities of daily living such as eating, bathing, toileting, transport, or other assistance

- Served in military at least 90 days, including one day during wartime, prior to the Gulf War

  - This does NOT mean you have to be injured

- More information is provided by visiting the website, or calling the telephone number provided below

> Amounts of Aid and Attendance maximums for 2021
>
> https://veteransfinancial.com/aid-and-attendance-main/

Housebound Benefit

This benefit is also an Enhanced Pension offered through the Veterans Administration, and also includes the **surviving spouse.** To qualify for this benefit, a person must be confined to their home due to a permanent disability. This benefit is *in addition* to the basic monthly pension allowance, and is also **tax-free.**

A person cannot receive both the Aid and Attendance Benefit and the Housebound Benefit at the same time.

Even if you do not qualify for basic pension benefits due to inability to meet income requirements, you may qualify for the Aid and Attendance or Housebound Benefit programs due to a more expanded income eligibility requirement.

You may also obtain more information on both the Aid or Attendance Program and the Housebound Program by entering the link below in the search area on YouTube.

https://youtu.be/3_U_Ki-QwB0

vba.va.gov

For general VA benefits. Then type in **Aid and Attendance** or **Housebound Benefit** into the search area for more detailed information on both benefits

(877) 294-6380 (contact number for **Aid and Attendance** and **Housebound** Enhanced Pension Benefits)

Discount License Plates for Purple Heart Recipients

- *Nine* states offer **FREE** plates and registration

- *Eighteen* states offer **FREE** plates and have normal registration fees

- The remaining states have a mixture of plate costs and registration fees

- To find out what your state offers:

  - Contact your local **Department of Motor Vehicles** and inquire

Check the website for other benefits:

purpleheart.org

Call **(703) 642-5360** ext. **120** for service program

(888) 668-1656 (National Headquarters number)

Please refer to:
LICENSE PLATES section (page 129) for more information on FREE or discounted license plates, including those for Disabled Veterans

Burial Benefits

Many veterans don't know all (or most) of the benefits they are entitled to—especially when it comes to their final resting place, and/or basic funeral expenses.

Basic highlights are listed below, so be sure to review them carefully so you are aware of the options available. All our veterans deserve the honor and respect a military funeral offers, and I know I speak for a grateful nation (myself included), when I say "thank you" in advance to those who served!

- **Funeral Director – Key Source of Information**

  - It is very important to have a copy of your **DD Form 214** (honorable discharge paper) handy. It is suggested you give a copy of this form to the funeral director in advance, and before you ever need it.

  - The funeral director can also provide answers to many of your questions so you are prepared.

  - The information and entitlements called out in this section are not the same for all services. There are burial restrictions based on rank, combat service, years in service, plot availability, and more.

  - The funeral director must have a copy of the **DD214** form to obtain the casket, flag, color guard, headstone, and suggest available resting places and any other benefits, should you require them.

  - It can take up to three months to receive a copy of the **DD214** form from the various services, so you must plan ahead.

  - Also, the funeral director may apply to the VA for money to cover some expenses depending on funeral home operational procedures. Cremations are also an option.

  - The easiest way to obtain a copy of the **DD214** is to go online and search for **DD214**.

  - Find the branch of service that pertains, and follow the instructions. Some services offer expedited delivery, depending how long ago the person served. It may still take weeks to obtain a copy of the discharge papers.

  - Another area of concern may be the medals. The **DD214** also lists the authorized medals, which may also be requested from the branch of service you served under.

  - The **DD214** also lists the highest rank and dates of service for the head stone.

- **Military Funeral Honors Ceremony / "Honoring Those Who Served"**—provided at request of family and included at no charge

  - Taps played at funeral site for veteran

- Folding and presenting the United States burial flag

- Presidential Memorial Certificate

- Government headstone or marker

- **Burial benefits for spouse and dependents** (can include parents) buried in a national cemetery include:

  - Burial with the veteran—in same plot

  - Perpetual care

  - Spouse or dependents name(s), date of birth and death inscribed on veteran's headstone at **no cost** to family

  - Spouse, minor child, and single adult child in some cases—may all be buried there even if the veteran is buried elsewhere

- **Funeral expenses**—amount paid by the VA depends on whether the veteran died in a VA hospital, outside a hospital, and / or if buried in a plot outside a national cemetery

- **Sources of information**

  - The funeral director will contact the proper support agencies to obtain your benefits. In most cases they are the only individuals who can make these requests.

  - **Example:** If a firing squad is unavailable, the funeral director will coordinate with local veteran groups for that service (which is **FREE**… however, a small donation is always appreciated).

  - Contact the VA directly for additional information. There may be more benefits you may be entitled to yet do not know you are entitled to.

  - Local American Legion/VFW (Veterans of Foreign Wars) – Members may be entitled to additional benefits.

  - Army, Navy, Air Force bases – contact the HQS and request assistance from the survivor assistance officer.

GI Bill (Higher Education Benefit)

The military offers **FREE** education to those who have served our country. There are certain rules, stipulations, and a designated amount of time a veteran must serve—in order to partake in this benefit.*

Family members (including a spouse and children) are also able to receive these benefits when certain criteria are met.

There are several options to choose from, including the VA education benefits through the post 9-11 GI Bill (Chapter 33)—which is this most common, and easiest to qualify for.

Payments and maximum amounts may be prorated based on your "eligibility percentage" if you are not eligible for the full percentage amount.

To qualify for benefits, 90 days of active service is required.

You may be able to qualify for:

- Tuition and fees
- Monthly housing allowance
- Stipend for books and supplies
- One-time Rural Benefit for some veterans
- Up to 36 months of benefits

Benefits expire in 15 years if service ended *before* January 1, 2013, and *never* expire if service ended *after* January 1, 2013 under the Forever GI Bill—Harry W. Comery Veterans Educational Assistance Act.

*Call the VA for more details.

Tutor.com: FREE tutoring for Military Families

Students from military families are eligible to **FREE 24/7** access to the online tutoring program when help or assistance is needed with homework or studying. This program is funded by the U.S. Department of Defense and Coast Guard Mutual Assistance.

A professional tutor is available whenever the need arises, and whenever the student needs help.

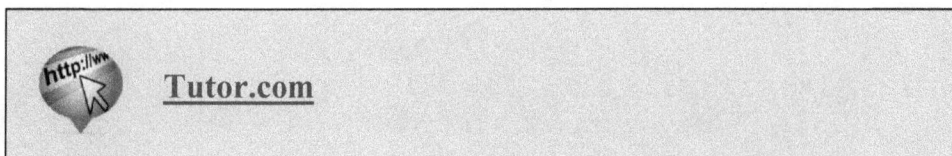

Tutor.com

Easter Seals

- Their objective is to assist children and adults with disabilities (**including veterans**) by providing medical and social services

- **Services:**

  - Medical rehabilitation

  - Respite care

  - Transportation solutions for caregivers

http://	**easterseals.com**
📱	(800) 221-6827 (312) 726-6200 (312) 726-1494 Fax
@	**info@easterseals.com**
MAIL	141 E. Jackson Blvd. # 1400 A Chicago, IL 60604

- Select **Our Programs** at the top of the page

  - Provides In-Home assistance

  - Provides respite care to the family caregiver

  - Employment services

  - Assistive technology

  - Childcare

  - Family support and veteran caregiver services

  - Camping programs for children

  - And much, much more...

Monty Roberts at "Flag Is Up Farms"

- Monty Roberts is known throughout the world for his violence-free method of horse training

- He has incorporated his methods in an equine assisted program for veterans suffering from symptoms of post-traumatic stress disorder (PTSD), with phenomenal results

- This three-day program is **FREE** to any veteran, and highly recommended

- For more information on the program, please contact the office at "Flag Is Up Farms," and ask about the **"Horse Sense and Healing Veterans Program"**

In the search area on YouTube.com type **"Veterans Thank Monty Roberts and the Horses"** OR **https://youtu.be/GaeiDRcG8LM** Hear directly from the veterans themselves who have taken the program. More videos are available both on YouTube.com & Monty's website below.

🌐	**join-up.org**
📱	(805) 688-6288
@	**admin@join-up.org** **info@montyroberts.com** (main office)
✉ MAIL	JOIN-UP INTERNATIONAL P.O. Box 246 Solvang, CA 93464

Military.com

- Website totally devoted to military personnel and veterans

- Information website for just about everything military

- Many **discounts** and **FREEBIES** available on this site (remember this resource guide primarily focuses on **FREE**, **deeply discounted**, or programs that offer **cash benefits**)

- Sign up for newsletter—receive additional special **discounts**

- Hover over the **Discounts** tab at the top right of the website, and select any of the links from the dropdown menu for **discounts** and **FREEBIES** of all kinds—including travel, theme parks, Disneyland, Disneyworld, museums, national parks, fitness clubs, restaurants, retail stores, and much more…

  - Always check the link "**Veterans Day Restaurant Discounts**" for **FREE meals** at a variety of restaurants on **Veterans Day**!

  - Restaurants like **Denny's** offer **15% veteran and senior discounts** every day of the week!

    - Other restaurants may offer everyday **discounts** as well

  - **Walmart** offers **20% discounts** on most items to active military and veterans

    - Other retailers may also offer everyday discounts as well

  - **Lowe's** and **Home Depot** offer a **10% discount** to active and reserve veterans, as well as those retired or disabled every day of the week

    - Other retailers may also offer everyday **discounts** as well

National Suicide Prevention Lifeline Hotline for Veterans

- Founded by the Department of Veterans Affairs

- Also known as "**Veterans Crisis Line**"

- Trained counselors take the calls—available 24 / 7

- **Please keep this number handy** should you or someone you love suffer from depression, suicidal thoughts, or PTSD

suicidepreventionlifeline.org

(800) 273-TALK (8255)
Press 1 to be routed to the Lifeline Hotline

PurpleHeart.org

- Has many links to explore and connect to benefit programs for **veterans**
- Some links on the site include:
  - Member benefits
    - Including local chapters
  - Suicide Awareness Program
  - Scholarship Program
  - POW / MIA Program
  - Homeless Veterans Program
  - Purple Heart Trail Program & more…

---

purpleheart.org

- Hover over **Our Services**
- From drop down menu a list of programs will appear

Wounded Warrior Project® (WWP)

- Created by Wounded Warriors for other Wounded Warriors
- Provides programs for caregivers and families of Wounded Warriors as well
- WWP Alumni offers many services beyond hospitalization, including an extensive Resource Center to help with all financial or physical needs of Warriors and their families (call the Resource Center number for more information)
- You MUST qualify as WWP Alumni to be eligible for services

Eligibility:

- You must have been injured (physical or psychological—stateside or deployed) on or after September 11, 2001 (Operation Enduring Freedom)

- May be eligible if you are the spouse or family member, and joining on behalf of a Warrior, and *if* the Warrior was injured *before*—but participated *in*—Operation Enduring Freedom or *after*

- You must then sign up as a WWP Alumni for services

- **Project Odyssey**

  - Brings fellow Warriors together dealing with combat stress disorder (physical and emotional stress)

  - Utilizes the power of nature and team-building exercises to recognize and adapt to stress

- **Coping and Family Service**

---

woundedwarriorproject.org

(904) 296-7350
(877) TEAMWWP (832-6997)
(888) 997-2586 (direct to the Resource Center)

Check the website for additional services that are available.
WWP is a VA-accredited organization and can help veterans with their VA claims.

MISCELLANEOUS ORGANIZATIONS / SERVICES

211

- Supported by the United Way and Alliance for Information and Referral Systems (AIRS)

- Provides information on local human services in your community including:

  - Training / Employment

  - Help paying bills

  - Food pantries

  - Help for an aging parent

  - Addiction prevention programs for teenage children

  - Affordable housing

  - Support groups

- Not available in all communities

- For additional information, see **page 113**.

---

211 websites by state

- To find your 211 state website:

- Type **"211 (your state) website"** into your browser

- **Examples**: "211 New York website," "211 Iowa website," "211 Texas website," etc.

- The 211 website for your state will appear with all the services they provide

211
This really is the number (like 911) where **local** help and assistance is available from your state

---

Johnson & Johnson Patient Assistance Foundation

- An independent nonprofit organization

- Helps the uninsured, those who have medications not covered by insurance, and those who are in financial need to be able to receive **FREE** medications donated by Johnson & Johnson Operating Companies (income requirements vary by medication)

- Forty prescription products available—select **Medications Available** tab at top of page to see if your medication is on the list

- Select **How to apply** tab (also at top of page) to see if you are eligible for the program

- May apply online if you meet the requirements

  OR

- **Call the 800 number** and have the application mailed or faxed to you

- You can also view a short **informative video** that explains the program and how to apply— select **About our programs** tab at the top of page to view

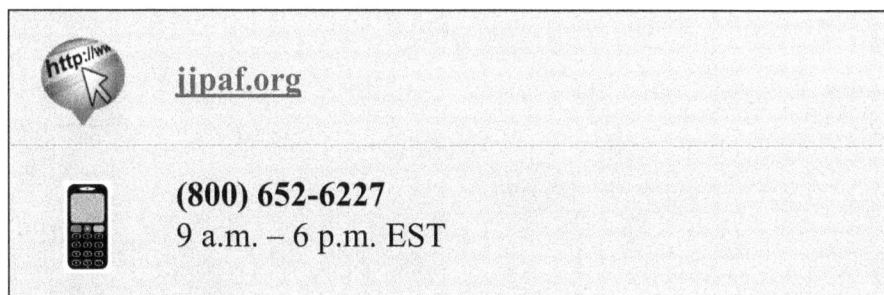

jjpaf.org

(800) 652-6227
9 a.m. – 6 p.m. EST

American Seniors Association (ASA)

- Another alternative to American Association of Retired Persons (AARP)

- No age minimum to join

- Membership cost $15 per year

- Membership benefits in areas of:

  - Security products

  - Financial

  - Insurance

  - Travel

- Health
- More...

americanseniors.org

(800) 951-0017

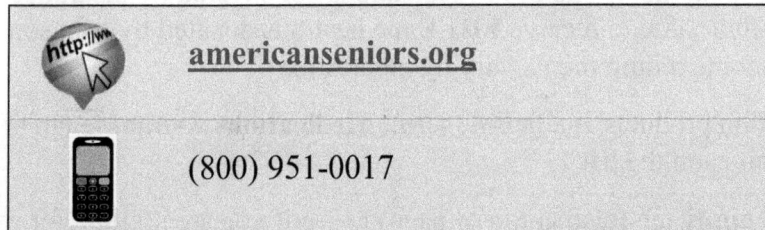

American Association of Retired Persons (AARP)

- Membership cost $16 per year and includes spouse or partner for **FREE** (Veterans are entitled to a 30% discount on membership)
- Must be over 55
- Numerous benefits in each of the following categories:
  - Health
  - **Discounts** (many discount area choices, including everyday purchases up to 60% off)
  - Travel
  - Financial
  - Insurance
  - Books, articles, online games
  - Extensive information to help caregivers
  - Local event dates and contact information
  - Much, much more...

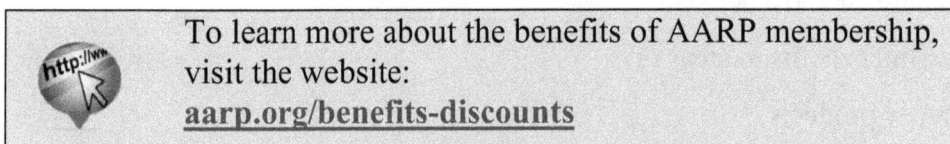

To learn more about the benefits of AARP membership, visit the website:
aarp.org/benefits-discounts

AARP offers a vast array of benefits besides those listed above. These benefits are far too numerous to mention, and cover many, many topics relevant to seniors and their needs.

http://	**AARP.org**
📱	**(888) 687-2277** 7 a.m. – 11 p.m. EST (Monday – Friday)

Benefits Check Up

- Benefits Check Up was developed and is maintained by the National Council on Aging (NCOA)
- Their website is very easy to navigate
- They provide assistance in the following areas:
  - Healthcare
  - Heating bills / utilities
  - Legal services
  - Meals / food assistance
  - Prescriptions
  - Taxes
  - Transportation
  - Employment training
  - In-Home services

http://	**benefitscheckup.org**
📱	National Council on Aging **(800) 794-6559** 9 a.m. – 5 p.m. EST (Monday – Friday)

Once you are on the website:

- At top of page select **Find My Benefits**
- You will then need to enter your **zip code** and select **Let's Get Started**
- Fill out all the information requested, then select **Get Results**

- Will provide a variety of programs and services available to you, based on how you answered the questions and your specific requests

- May be some overlapping and similarities with information found on other websites—many programs and services do not always show up on every website

- Important to gather as much information as possible to have access to ALL options available

Caregiver Action Network (CAN)

- This website focuses on increasing the quality of life for caregivers by providing support, resources, and education regarding every aspect of caring for a loved one.

- This website is easy to navigate, has practical and useful information in many areas of interest, has a forum, and easy to access to just about anything by topic.

You can always refer to this site later if you are currently pressed for time. However, the **'Medicare'** video listed at the top of the next page, and the **'Video Series-Alzheimer's Caregivers' (VSAC),** are both worth watching. The VSAC is a series of short videos on just about every aspect of caregiving, not just Alzheimer's. The 'Medicare' webinar and the 'Video Series-Alzheimer's Caregivers' are found when you select the **Toolbox** tab at the top of the page, then select the appropriate blue boxes to view the titles or topics you are looking for.

The **Agencies & Organizations** link on the left side of the Toolbox page also provides many valuable contacts that are caregiver specific.

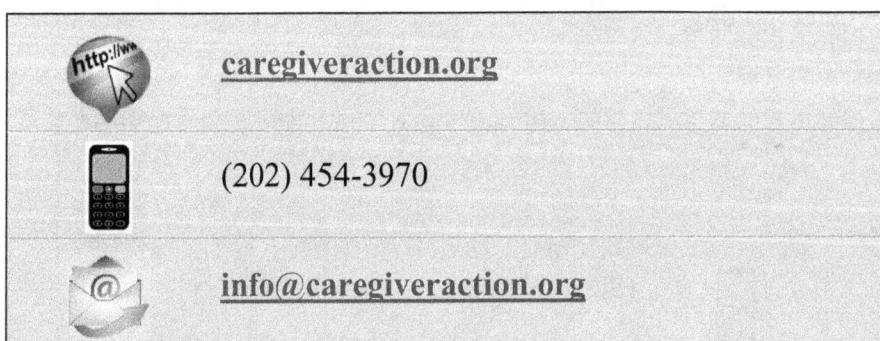

http://w	caregiveraction.org
📱	(202) 454-3970
@	info@caregiveraction.org

Is Medicare a bit confusing and difficult to understand?

Go to the website **caregiveraction.org.** Select the **Toolbox** tab at the top of the page, then select the blue box that says **"Video Series-Understanding Medicare."**

This video series provides one of the **BEST** explanations regarding all aspects of Medicare. It is presented in short, bite sized, easy to understand segments, with graphics and visuals to help explain each area. A **MUST** watch!

Elder Care Locator

- Eldercare Locator is a nationwide **FREE** public service funded by the U.S. Administration on Aging

- Helps seniors and caregivers find local agencies in every U.S. Community

- This website is very easy to navigate—all local contact information is provided

eldercare.acl.gov

- Under **Find Help in Your Community** enter **zip code** or **city and state**

- Select the **Search** tab

- Provides information from a list of services available

(800) 677-1116

9 a.m. – 6 p.m. EST (Monday – Friday)

Note: When you fill in your **zip code** or **city**, it will bring up a list of the Area Agencies on Aging in your local area (including all phone numbers, contact information, and breakdown of services and programs they provide), and other contacts. You may already have some of the local numbers. Check the list to see if you may have missed anything.

Easter Seals

The objective of Easter Seals is to assist children and adults with disabilities (**including veterans**) by providing medical and social services.

easterseals.com

	(800) 221-6827 (312) 726-6200 (312) 726-1494 Fax
	info@easterseals.com
	141 E. Jackson Blvd. # 1400 A Chicago, IL 60604

- At the top of the page under **Our Programs** find information for:
  - **AUTISM**
    - o Provides a variety of services for both children and adults
  - **VETERANS / VETERAN REINTEGRATION**
    - o Provides In-Home assistance
    - o Provides respite care to the family caregiver
    - o Employment services
    - o Assistive technology
    - o Childcare
    - o Family support
    - o Camping programs for children
    - o And much, much more...
  - **CHILDREN & YOUNG ADULT SERVICES**
    - o Helps children & young adults with disabilities
    - o Aides in special healthcare needs
  - **ADULT, SENIOR, & CAREGIVER SERVICES**
    - o Adult day care services
    - o In-Home support and services
    - o Medical rehabilitation
    - o Community mobility options

- Wellness programs

- Support and respite services for family caregivers

- Senior transportation to help keep them independent

- Transportation solutions for caregivers

- Many services for caregivers

- **MEDICAL REHABILITATION**

  - Offers a variety of assistance to children and adults, including speech, physical and occupational therapy, hearing, and more

Family Caregiver Alliance®: National Center on Caregiving

This is an *excellent* website that offers a wealth of information, classes, webinars, videos, research, support groups, products, and more, including **Disease-Specific Organizations (DSO)** available in each state. Keep in mind there may be other DSO resources available in your state that are not listed on this website, and each state varies.

Please make a note to investigate this website thoroughly, as it will provide information that is easy to access, and will help answer many of your questions on a variety of topics.

For more specific programs and resources in *your* state, follow the links below.

> **caregiver.org**
>
> - Find the map
>
> - **Select your state** for a list of resources, programs, and information
>
> - Resources also include **Disease-Specific Organizations**

FREE Legal Help for Seniors

- **Contact your local Office for the Aging**

  - Type in **"Office for the Aging (your city and state)"** OR **"FREE Legal Help for Seniors"**

    - **Example:** "Office for the Aging Clearwater, Florida" OR "FREE Legal Help for Seniors"

- Various alternative names may appear (like Area Agency on Aging, etc.)

- **Call your local office**—ask for local law school that has a Senior Law Center specifically for low income seniors

  o Instrumental with drafting a simple will, certifying a Power of Attorney (POA) or healthcare proxy, or drafting a letter to creditors

  o If local Office for the Aging is unaware of local resources offering this help, contact your local Lions Club

  o Many Lions Club members are attorneys, and can help find a pro bono attorney to help you

---

LionsClubs.org

Lions Club International

(630) 571-5466
(ask for contact information to local Lions Club)

LifeLine

- Is a federal government assistance program

- Provides one **FREE** or discounted phone (landline or cell phone) per household

  OR

- Provides discount on phone bill

- Seniors and other qualified individuals must be on some form of government assistance

  - Food Stamps

  - Supplemental Security Income

  - Federal Public Housing Assistance

  - Tribal Programs (and live on Tribal Lands)

  - Medicaid

  - Veterans Pension or Survivors Benefits

- $9.25 phone bill credit given—up to extra $25 additional credit given to Tribal LifeLine

- Check with your local phone provider to see if they are on the list of providers

- Check **LifeLinesupport.org** links on left side of page to find:

  - Companies near you

  - Do you qualify?

  - Documents needed

  - How to apply

  - More…

http://w	**LifeLinesupport.org**
📱	(800) 234-9473

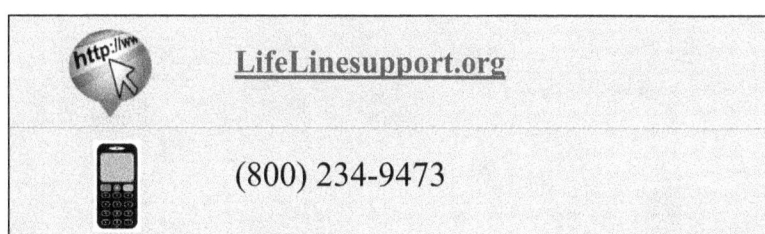

Medical Equipment Loaned Out

There are many places that actually lend out medical equipment for **FREE**.

- Type in **"medical equipment to lend out (your city and state)"** in the address bar of your browser

  - Will bring up list of places that lend out medical equipment for **FREE**

- **Examples:**

  - **"medical equipment to lend out Washington, DC"**

  - **"medical equipment to lend out Philadelphia, PA"**

National Volunteer Caregiving Network

- The primary goal of this program is to provide assistance to homebound neighbors with chronic health conditions or disabilities

- Available in many areas of the country

- Provides assistance in the following non-medical areas:

  - Shopping

  - Reading

- Bill payment
- Minor home repairs
- Light housework
- Transportation to medical and other appointments
- Respite care
- Visiting and companionship

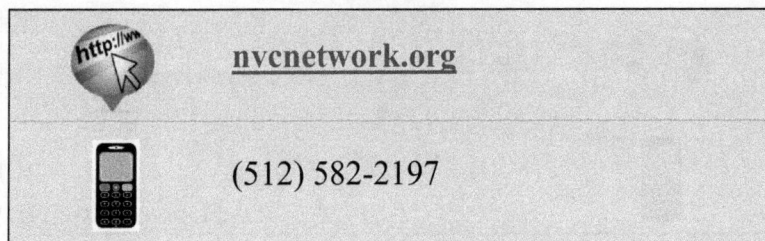

nvcnetwork.org

(512) 582-2197

Select the **Find a Program Near You** tab at the top of the page.

Enter **zip code, city,** or **state** in the **"query"** field above the map.

Select **Find a Volunteer Caregiver** located below the map.

Fill out the requested information.

Select the **Send Request** button and someone will contact you within three business days.

Please feel free to also call the number above for further assistance. They will be more than happy to assist you.

Senior Discounts (FREE or Discounted)

When you become an elite member of the 55+ Club… there are a variety of **FREE or discounted** products and services you now have the pleasure to partake in. Always remember to ask for them, because they may not be offered otherwise.

Businesses are often reluctant to offer these discounts to patrons NOT because they don't want to give them to you—but because some individuals may look older than their years, and may become offended if they are mistaken for being members of this elite group before their time. ☺

Places that often give discounts are listed below, so don't be afraid to ask for them.

AARP members are often given additional **discounts** with membership.

- Restaurants

- Movie theaters (**FREE** admission often given to caregivers accompanying person in wheelchair)

- Hotels / Motels

- Theme Parks / National Parks

- Fitness Centers

- Travel (airlines, busses, trains)

- **FREE or discounted** tuition to universities. Type in "**what states offer FREE tuition to seniors**" in the address bar of your browser for a list of universities offering **FREE** or **discounted** tuition

- Online retailers

- Prescriptions (see **Prescription Section** of this Resource Guide)

- License plates (see **License Plate Section** of this Resource Guide)

- Dental services (**DentalLifeline.org**)

- Legal services (**ElderCare.acl.gov**)

- Food (see **FOOD Section** of this Resource Guide)

SeniorsFirst.org (California Only)

- A nonprofit organization that is a great resource for caregivers seeking services for a senior loved one

- Services Placer County, California ONLY

- Programs include:

  - Transportation – My Rides (FREE non-emergency medical and non-medical appointments)

  - Adult Day Programs

  - Caregiver counseling & support services / Information & Assistance

  - Friendly visitor program

  - Living Placement – Out-of-home living situations

  - Transportation – Health Express (non-emergency medical appointments)

  - Senior nutrition programs

http://w	**seniorsfirst.org**
📱	**(800) 878-9222** (Seniors First/Meals on Wheels)

FREE Walkers or Rollators

- Hospitals and nursing homes often dispose of reliable used medical equipment
  - Check periodically with these places to check if they have walkers or other used medical equipment available for **FREE**
  - Places like Goodwill and various Thrift Shops often have reliable used medical equipment for reasonable prices

United Way

- Check with your local United Way chapter to inquire regarding services they may offer
  - Housekeeping services
  - Respite care for caregivers
  - Directions for food pantries in your area
  - **FREE** or **reduced** dental programs

http://w	**unitedway.org** Select the link **Find Your United Way** at top right of the page Enter **zip code** and submit for contact information in your area
📱	**(703) 836-7112** 8:30 a.m. – 6:30 p.m. EST (Monday – Friday)

CHECKLISTS FOR BENEFICIAL RESOURCES

DENTAL SERVICES

Note: *Author grants permission for you to make copies of this checklist for your future needs and as your information changes.*

NAME of LOCAL PROGRAM	
📱	
http://w	
CONTACT PERSON	
Dates called:	
PRICES	$
	$
	$

EYECARE

Note: *Author grants permission for you to make copies of this checklist for your future needs and as your information changes.*

NAME of LOCAL PROGRAM	
CONTACT PERSON	
Dates called:	
PRICES	$
	$
	$

FOOD RESOURCES

Note: *Author grants permission for you to make copies of this checklist for your future needs and as your information changes.*

NAME of LOCAL PROGRAM	
📱	
🌐	
CONTACT PERSON	
Dates called:	

ENERGY ASSISTANCE

Note: *Author grants permission for you to make copies of this checklist for your future needs and as your information changes.*

NAME of LOCAL PROGRAM	
CONTACT PERSON	
Dates called:	

FUNERAL RESOURCES

Note: *Author grants permission for you to make copies of this checklist for your future needs and as your information changes.*

COMPANY NAME	
📱	
🌐	
CONTACT PERSON	
Dates called:	
PRICES	$
	$
	$

DISCOUNT LICENSE TAGS

Note: *Author grants permission for you to make copies of this checklist for your future needs and as your information changes.*

SECRETARY of STATE / DEPARTMENT of MOTOR VEHICLES in *your state*	
QUALIFICATIONS	
CONTACT PERSON	
Dates called:	
DISCOUNT AMOUNT	$

PRESCRIPTION DISCOUNT PLAN

Note: *Author grants permission for you to make copies of this checklist for your future needs and as your information changes.*

PLAN NAME	
📱	
🌐	
CONTACT PERSON	
Dates called:	
DISCOUNT AMOUNT	$
Generic Medications:	

Note: *Author grants permission for you to make copies of this checklist for your future needs and as your information changes.*

Make a list of all your medications, their strengths, & how often you take them.

MEDICATION	STRENGTH (Dose)	FREQUENCY (How often it's taken)	#Tablets / Vials Used per Month
Pharmacies that have my generic medications for $4 – $10:			

RESPITE CARE AGENCY

Note: *Author grants permission for you to make copies of this checklist for your future needs and as your information changes.*

AGENCY NAME	
CONTACT PERSON	
QUALIFICATIONS:	
Dates called:	
PRICES:	$
	$
	$

NUTRITIONAL SUPPLEMENTS

Note: *Author grants permission for you to make copies of this checklist for your future needs and as your information changes.*

COMPANY NAME	
CONTACT PERSON	
Dates called:	
PRICES:	$ $ $

VETERANS' BENEFITS

Note: *Author grants permission for you to make copies of this checklist for your future needs and as your information changes.*

PROGRAM NAME	
📱	
🌐	
CONTACT PERSON	
QUALIFICATIONS:	
Dates called:	
Benefits received: (make sure you also obtain your DD214 form to receive full benefits)	

THERAPY ANIMALS / SERVICE ANIMALS

Note: *Author grants permission for you to make copies of this checklist for your future needs and as your information changes.*

PROGRAM NAME	
CONTACT PERSON	
QUALIFICATIONS:	
Dates called:	
Wait time for animal:	

DISABILITY RESOURCES

Note: *Author grants permission for you to make copies of this checklist for your future needs and as your information changes.*

PROGRAM NAME	
📱	
http://www	
CONTACT PERSON	
QUALIFICATIONS:	
Dates called:	
Other information:	

OTHER PROGRAMS IN YOUR AREA

Note: *Author grants permission for you to make copies of this checklist for your future needs and as your information changes.*

PROGRAM NAME	
CONTACT PERSON	
QUALIFICATIONS:	
Dates called:	
Services provided:	

OTHER PROGRAMS IN YOUR AREA

Note: *Author grants permission for you to make copies of this checklist for your future needs and as your information changes.*

PROGRAM NAME
CONTACT PERSON
QUALIFICATIONS:
Dates called:
Services provided:

OTHER PROGRAMS IN YOUR AREA

Note: *Author grants permission for you to make copies of this checklist for your future needs and as your information changes.*

PROGRAM NAME
CONTACT PERSON
QUALIFICATIONS:
Dates called:
Services provided:

FINANCIAL HOUSEKEEPING

"Yesterday is a cancelled check.
Today is cash on the line.
Tomorrow is a promissory note."
—Hank Stram

FINANCIAL REALITIES

For the most part, birth is seen as a joyous and happy time. There are baby showers, planning for the new arrival, and the air is filled with expectancy, hope, and excitement.

The aging process and the subject of death often do not share the same enthusiasm.

The latter years are often spent in financial desperation due to illness, lack of planning for the "golden years," or simply not knowing what to do when the unexpected happens.

While financial planning may be confusing, complicated, or overwhelming, it is extremely important and necessary to consider.

It may seem unpleasant to put final paperwork in order, yet without proper strategies in place, a large portion of your hard-earned money will be unnecessarily eaten up by expenses.

Advanced financial planning provides protection of your assets and comfort to loved ones in the times of distress.

It is also important to have all papers, contact information, and locations of important documents in a place where they are easy to access—and making sure at least two trusted individuals know where these documents are located.

There is a checklist available at the end of this section to help and assist you with this task.

CURRENT RATES OF CARE

Nursing Home

- $245+ per day (national average) for semi-private room

- $275+ per day (national average) for private room

- $8,517 per month (national average) for private room

- $7,441 per month (national average) per month for semi-private room

Note: *These rates do not include any special services. Residents with dementia, Alzheimer's, ventilation needs, and other special services, will incur additional charges.*

Assisted Living Facility

- $132 per day (national average)

- $4,051 per month (national average) for a one bedroom unit

In-Home Nurse (through an agency)

- On average, the rate for a licensed practical nurse (LPN) is $40 per hour weekdays and $45 per hour on weekends, with a 40 hour work-week commitment, and can cost up to $75 per hour

- For 'as needed' care, there is a two hour minimum for anything less than two hours, $80 for two hours on weekdays, and a $90 minimum on weekends

- Many agencies require a four hour minimum

Home Health Aide

- Each state varies regarding services, and whether you choose to go through an agency (higher rate) or private hire (lower rate)

- Rates may vary from $21 – $23 per hour (national average), depending on the state

- $4,385 per month (national average)

- $183,456 per year, private homecare at $21 per hour 24/7

- Having to hire someone just three times per week, will bring the cost of services to approximately $22,000 per year (on average)

A great way to protect your hard earned money from these astronomical charges is to obtain Long Term Care Insurance BEFORE you need it!

LONG-TERM CARE INSURANCE

Long-Term Care (LTC) Insurance is a relatively new type of insurance. Originally, it was introduced in the 1980s to cover nursing home expenses. However, the insurance policies have changed, and it now covers much more than it did originally.

Depending on the type of LTC insurance purchased, a person may begin collecting on the policy when assistance is needed for two or more activities of daily living. Several examples of these activities of daily living may include bathing, clothing, feeding, and toilet assistance.

Statistics show that 35% of people over 65 years of age will need some type of nursing home care in their lifetime. One person in seven will be disabled five or more years before retiring.

Long-term care insurance helps protect some of the assets a person acquired over his or her lifetime.

Some of the services that may be covered:

- Nursing home care
- Home healthcare
- Personal care in home
- Services in assisted living facilities
- Services in adult day care centers

Advantages of Long Term Care Insurance:

- You *can* be treated at home
- Covers a majority of expenses
- Decreases the financial burden on you and your family

It is advisable to speak to an insurance agent to help decide if LTC insurance is something that would be beneficial to you, including what services are available and covered under the policy.

Age is another factor to consider. The younger you are, the less your monthly premiums. Costs are based on other variables as well, and must be purchased prior to actually needing the insurance.

Research the viability of your LTC insurance company. You will want an insurance company that will be around in 20 years if, and when, you need to use the insurance.

There is much to consider when choosing a policy. Take the time to review the options, as both the cost and length of service in years will vary, depending on the policy chosen.

Most LTC insurance policies do not pay family members who give 'in-home' care.

TRUST VERSUS WILL

Whether or not there is a plan in place for the cost of care, obtaining a Trust is vitally important. There must be some financial documentation in place to avoid probate from obtaining a substantial chunk of the estate.

Without a Trust, probate can very easy drain huge amounts of cash from the estate. These expenditures are hidden in attorney fees, court costs, executor fees, and whatever else is deemed necessary.

A Will does not avoid probate. Probate holds the estate open for 4 to 14 months (or years), allowing challenges to the estate. Therefore, it is essential to have something in place before the person dies.

All Wills still pass through probate. Attorneys may charge from 3% to 11% of the estate just for representation in Probate Court. All fees mentioned previously may be added to the cost. Anything that goes through probate becomes public record. Therefore, with only a Will in place, anyone may discover personal information about the size of the estate and other private matters.

A Living Trust may be drawn up by anyone, regardless of how many or how few assets they may have. A Living Trust has many benefits. Some of the advantages are listed below.

Advantages of a Living Trust When a Person Is Alive

- Complete control over the entire estate is maintained

- Can be structured to provide management of assets to ensure the holder of the trust is taken care of in the future, should they be unable to manage them when they are older

- To take advantage of the benefits of a trust, a person must transfer all titles of assets into the trust

Advantages of a Living Trust Upon Death

- Does not have to go through probate

- Funds are available to heirs immediately after the person's death without any court proceedings

- It is more difficult for a disgruntled heir to contest a Living Trust as opposed to a Will

- A Living Trust is not public record

- Charity donations designated in a Living Trust cannot be reduced by heirs to the estate

It is imperative that legal council is received regarding any financial affairs—ensuring everything is in order. If you wish to set up a Living Trust, please seek another opinion if you are told that a Will is all that is necessary to protect assets.

Remember, a Will must still go through probate. Attorneys are entitled to collect a fee unless other arrangements have been made in advance.

Laws continue to change, and there are many attorneys who specialize in Trusts, Elder Care, and Elder Law. Therefore, it is vitally important to speak to an attorney who is familiar with the most current laws. Many attorneys are very well versed on the needs of the elderly. In fact, you may already know a good attorney who is. If you currently do not have an attorney you know and trust, you may wish to contact the National Academy of Elder Law Attorneys.

The National Academy of Elder Law Attorneys (NAELA)

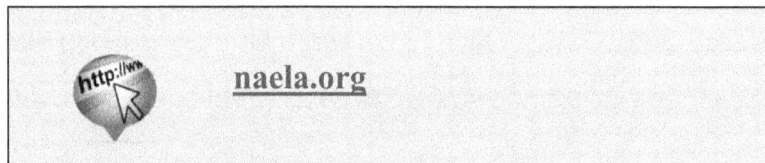

naela.org

NAELA attorneys are composed of professionals who deal with legal issues affecting seniors and people with disabilities as they age.

To find an Elder Law Attorney, select the large red rectangle to the left of the page that says, **Find a Lawyer.**

Enter your **city** and **state** and the **distance in miles** you wish to travel, and a list of Elder Law Attorneys in your area will appear.

Please review this site, as you will find all the latest legislation, events, and a wealth of information regarding the elderly.

An attorney should be able to give legal counsel on:

Transferring of Assets

- Ask what time-frame is mandatory in your state for transferring assets to become qualified for Medicaid

- Most states, but not all, are adopting the 60-month rule (five years)

- In Michigan for example, in order for assets to be protected and not be taken by Medicaid (to cover a person's care), the assets must be transferred five years prior to qualifying for eligibility

Power of Attorney / Durable Power of Attorney

- A legal document that appoints a person of your choice to make decisions on your behalf should you become incapacitated and unable to make decisions for yourself

- Must be in place before you become incapacitated to be valid—consult with attorney for more details

Advance Directive

- A document that allows you to outline provisions about your future medical care, should you be unable to speak for yourself due to a serious illness or incapacitation

Critical decisions will be made for you by institutions, health care providers, or a court appointed guardian, if an Advance Directive or a Durable Power of Attorney is not in place.

- Must be in place before you become incapacitated to be valid—consult with attorney for more details

Guardianship / Conservatorship

- A court appointed person who manages the personal finances and healthcare of someone who is unable to do these tasks on their own

  - This court appointed person is chosen when the individual failed to draw up a Durable Power of Attorney and / or an Advance Directive prior to becoming incapacitated

- Guardianship has more power than a Power of Attorney in decision-making and direct accessibility to the person's personal records, medical history, and medical records

- Having Guardianship can be vitally important regarding major decisions that must often be made on issues of importance

CHECKLIST FOR VITAL / FINANCIAL INFORMATION

Note: *Author grants permission for you to make copies of this checklist for your future needs and as your information changes.*

FINANCIAL INFORMATION

Company / Institution and account numbers	
ACCOUNT	ACCOUNT NUMBER
Life Insurance	

Disability Insurance	

Credit card numbers	

Checking	

Savings	

CDs	

Mutual Funds	

Stocks & Bonds	

SAFE / SAFETY DEPOSIT BOX

SAFE	
Location	
Combination	
Location	
Combination	

SAFETY DEPOSIT BOX	
Box location	
Key location	
Cosigner(s)	
Box location	
Key location	
Cosigner(s)	

ATTORNEY	
Name	
Address	
Telephone(s)	
Email	

ACCOUNTANT	
Name	
Address	
Telephone(s)	
Email	

BROKER	
Name	
Address	
Telephone(s)	
Email	

CLERGY	
Name	
Address	
Telephone(s)	
Email	

PRIMARY CARE PHYSICIAN	
Name	
Address	
Telephone(s)	
Email	

Obtain a copy of the Trust / Will

- Keep the original in the safe deposit box
- Make several other notarized copies and place a copy in a designated area where you and someone you trust can easily access it
- Location(s):_____

Copy of Advance Directive

- Include **DO NOT RESUSCITATE** (DNR) papers, should you choose this option
    - These are either 8½" x 11" or wallet sized, signed by the physician, and generally printed on **bright colored** paper

Copy of Power of Attorney

Copy of conservatorship papers (if needed)

Deed / title to the home and any other additional land / properties

Social Security Number:_____

Copy of marriage license / divorce papers

Copy of birth certificate

Military service information:

Branch of Service: _____

Military ID # _____

Dates of Service: _____

Copy of form DD 214: _____

Burial information

Funeral home: _____

Copy of form DD 214 given to funeral director for military funeral: _____

All information necessary for a military funeral / military funeral arrangements
(**see page 182** for more details)_____

Church service: _____

Cemetery information / location:_____

EMOTIONAL CARE

"Always reach for a better feeling thought!"

—Abraham Hicks

IMPACT OF CAREGIVING

Depression

Family caregivers, especially those that have been actively involved in this role for an extended period of time, are very prone to depression.

You, as a caregiver, may not even realize how depressed you may be because you are so busy with daily caregiving responsibilities. Signs of depression may be vague, so they are often overlooked or dismissed. For this reason, many caregivers do not associate depression with any or all of the symptoms listed below.

Some signs of depression to watch for:

- Lack of energy, feeling constantly drained and fatigued
- Decreased interest in self (are you wearing sweatpants or scrubs every day and forgetting to shower?)
- Feelings of isolation
- Not doing things that used to bring joy
- Easily agitated
- Change in eating habits (weight gain or loss)
- Change in sleep pattern (either too little or excessive sleeping)
- Loss of self-esteem
- Feeling hopeless and helpless
- Avoiding social contact
- Inability to concentrate and focus

Facts:

- The rate of depression is higher in women than in men
- Approximately 12 million women experience clinical depression each year—double that of men
- Women provide the majority of caregiving—40% of men are now caregivers

I cannot stress enough how vitally important it is to take care of yourself. I know you have probably heard this many times before. Now you are hearing it again from me.

So why is caring for yourself so important?

Caregiving is more hazardous to your health than you may realize, especially if you don't know what to do to help yourself. Statistics are stacked against you emotionally, physically, and from a general health standpoint. Be aware of the subtle changes taking place in your life every single day.

Catching the symptoms early is also beneficial. These symptoms may cascade into a downward spiral of clinical depression, which is far more severe.

If you are a woman experiencing signs of menopause or perimenopause, also consider your hormones are most likely out of balance. This imbalance may also be contributing to your depression, and it may be time to consult with a physician or holistic practitioner.

You may already know that depression can be paralyzing and life altering. It is not something to be taken lightly, so please seek professional help and advice should these symptoms persist.

Did you know:

- 'Negative ions' are important for overall health and wellness because they enhance mood, purify the air, remove pollen, allergens, other airborne particles, and more...

- Moving water is a natural producer of negative ions

  - This is why you feel more energized, positive, and refreshed after a rainstorm, around bodies of moving water (like an ocean or waterfall, for example), or after taking a shower

- Taking a shower will increase your mood, mental clarity, and sense of well-being, because moving water helps generate negative ions

- If you feel depressed or a little low on energy, think about taking a shower (and don't forget to wash your hair!)

- A 'Negative Ion Generator' may be purchased from local or online merchants, and is able to fill a room with negative ions. These negative ions attach to, and reduce, airborne particles that help keep the air energized and clean while promoting a sense of well-being.

At the end of this section, please read the information on Dehydration and Full-Spectrum Lighting. Both may contribute to depression and fatigue.

Both topics will offer valuable information, as well as interesting reading!

Statistics of Caregivers

The following statistics pertain to caregivers in general. You may not be aware of these statistics, and they are included here for you to review only. The list is even more extensive than you might imagine, and far too long to include everything in this section.

- There is a 63% higher mortality rate in elderly spousal caregivers (who have a history of chronic illness themselves) who experience stress directly related to caregiving, compared to those of their non-caregiving peers

- The stress of caring for a person with dementia has been shown to impact a family caregiver up to three years after the caregiving ends. This means all the time you are caring for a loved one, and up to three years after the care stops, you have an increased risk of developing a chronic illness yourself

- If you are caring for your spouse, you are six times more likely to experience anxiety or depression—if you are caring for your parent, you are twice as likely to experience these emotions

- If you are a husband caring for your wife, her hospitalization increases your mortality risk by 35% within a month

- Extreme stress has shown to age family caregivers, taking as much as ten years off their lives

- As a family caregiver, you have more than twice the rate of having a chronic illness than those who are non-caregivers, and 30% of all caregivers die before those they care for

Often, the caregiving responsibility falls on one member of the family. This person may be you.

If family members observe you are doing a good job, they will often simply allow you continue, as they may have no idea what you may be going through. They may not realize how physically tired or how mentally drained you may be, unless you go out of your way to tell them.

As difficult as it might be for you to do, you must ask for help! Having any kind of help and assistance is crucial to prevent burnout, stress, and physical health issues down the road.

Caring for yourself *first* is crucial if you are to be effective in caring for someone else. You may be thinking, *"Yeah, right. Who has time to really DO that?!"*

For starters, if you make *anything* a priority, it somehow always gets done.

Now is a good time for a change of mindset!

Repeat the following:

- ***I am important!***

- ***I cannot take care of anyone until I take care of myself first!***

Very Personal Note from Camille:

Caregivers often become ill within three years of any type of long-term caregiving.

For me, my entire body and immune system shut down within one month following my mother's death. I was unable to speak for 10½ months due to paralyzed vocal cords—and a compromised immune system brought its own set of 'goodies.'

Painful joints and muscles became daily visitors, along with chronic fatigue and excessive weight gain. I didn't realize how depressed I was, until I began to return to normal.

Looking back... I often wonder how I made it through every day.

Remember something extremely important... Although we might not be able to change circumstances, we can change how we choose to get through them. I only wish I knew then what I know now!

Most caregivers think they are "supermen" or "superwomen," thinking they are able to juggle multiple tasks at once, only to discover this caregiving thing is a mighty big job. I don't know why, but many of us seem to go through this "superperson" syndrome, only to suffer as a result.

So pause for a moment... take a breath... and acknowledge this fact.

Asking for help is not a weakness... it's a matter of survival! Please take what I say to heart, as I, too, had to learn the hard way. If you are a new caregiver, you may not realize how quickly your health may become compromised. When that happens, you will be of no use to anyone.

And always remember you are not alone! This was a concept I learned only after the death of both parents, and after I started my Caregiver page on Facebook (Caregiver Resource Inc).

By hearing from others, I realized how many of us all thought the same things, and often felt isolated and alone. It was only after my caregiving experience, I realized we caregivers belong to a very special and extraordinary group.

We've gone through the trenches, kept strong when we felt weak, kept going when we wanted to quit, had hope when others gave up, and somehow always managed to muster up courage we didn't know we possessed.

Not everyone is able to do what we do!

So, start today by taking better care of yourself, and know you are not alone. We are all bound together by the strongest cord in the world—the cord of LOVE—and this bond can only be shared and understood by a fellow comrade.

No words have to be spoken, because we have privately shared so much.

God Bless you and thank you for being part of my "family!"

Other Factors that May Contribute to Depression and Fatigue

Dehydration

Water is the essential essence of life. Without it, we would all perish.

Water helps flush toxins from the body, keeps the tissues hydrated, and maintains blood pressure. Therefore, it is essential to make it a priority to consume enough water every single day to keep our bodies healthy and vibrant.

This is especially true for seniors and the elderly.

Besides consuming water for physical health reasons, lack of hydration may also contribute to depression and fatigue.

An interesting and inexpensive way to prove this is to pay careful attention to how you feel when adequate amounts of water aren't consumed every day. Keep a journal and document everything. You will soon see the value of staying hydrated.

Drink the purest water possible. A good filtration system will also help to improve the taste. The better the taste, the easier it will be to drink.

When you are properly hydrated, you rarely (if ever) feel thirsty.

Make sure you consult with your healthcare professional to determine the proper amount of water you should be drinking every day.

Signs of dehydration:

- Dry skin
- Skin on the back of the hand does not immediately snap back when you pinch it
- Dry mouth
- Excessive thirst
- Depression, lack of clear thinking
- Fatigue

Sunlight

Vitamin D is absorbed by the body from natural sunlight. Research has also shown that the sun provides more benefits than simply supplying vitamin D.

Seasonal Affective Disorder (SAD)

- Seasonal Affective Disorder (SAD) is a mood disorder sometimes referred to as the "winter blues"

- In the winter when there is less sunlight, people with otherwise normal mental health become affected

- Symptoms may include decreased energy and increased depression

Full-spectrum light therapy is very effective in treating SAD, and was made popular by Dr. John Ott, a pioneer in the field of full-spectrum lighting (natural sunlight).

When natural sunlight is not readily available during the winter months, full-spectrum light bulbs become a healthy and effective alternative.

About Dr. John Ott

- A pioneer in the field of full-spectrum lighting (natural sunlight)

- Famous for his work in time-lapse photography for Walt Disney

- Stumbled upon plants needing full-spectrum lighting for proper function

- Depending on the light wavelength that was 'missing'...

  - Plants would not mature

  - Buds would not fully bloom

  - Buds would fall off prematurely

  - And more...

- Dr. Ott went on to study animals by eliminating various wavelengths from full-spectrum light, and / or adding low level radiation (as from a television set), and noticed the following:

  - Loss of hair / fur

  - Problems with tail development or loss of tail

  - Obesity

  - Increased cholesterol

- Cancer

- Depression

- Agitation

- Aggression

- Decreased eye integrity

- Lack of general overall wellness

- He then turned his focus to humans—monitoring the benefits full-spectrum lighting had on them—and noticed that full-spectrum lighting *reduced* the following:

  - Hyperactivity in classrooms

  - Negative behaviors in prisons

  - Negative behaviors in mental health facilities

  - Absenteeism in the workplace

  - Incidences of illness

- Dr. Ott discovered that the individual cell's ability to properly reproduce in animals (including humans), was affected by light as it entered the body through the *eyes*!

  - Dr. Ott was not an advocate of traditional sunglasses

  - Colored lenses block certain wavelengths of light from entering the eyes

Please explore the resources below to find more information regarding Dr. Ott and his research regarding full-spectrum lighting.

I highly recommend you view some of John Ott's original time-lapse photography on YouTube.

The link to the YouTube video is included below, and also the *name* of the video—should you choose to type it in the search box.

- Go to: **YouTube.com**

  - In the search box on YouTube type in: **"John Ott – Exploring the Spectrum,"** Dr. John Ott documentary on the health effects of light

  OR

  - The link to the YouTube video below will also connect you to the material: https://youtu.be/BOUA8UAEAdY

  - Either way, you will be able to access this absolutely incredible video, and be able to watch the documentation of many of Dr. Ott's findings

John N. Ott's book, *Health and Light: The Extraordinary Study that Shows How Light Affects Your Health and Emotional Well-Being*—reveals research results on full-spectrum versus florescent light or other lighting that is not full-spectrum. These results confirmed that without full-spectrum lighting, plants were unable to reproduce successfully, and both animals and humans developed a variety of physical and emotional maladies.

While we may know there are dangers when we are overexposed to the sun's rays for extended periods, this must be tempered by the need for the full spectrum of light the same sun provides. Sunlight is essential to our well-being, as you will see from Dr. Ott's research. Small daily amounts are all you need, which is especially important during the winter months.

Through the research compiled from Dr. Ott's work, the **Ott Lite**® was invented, and it provides full-spectrum lighting in the home or office with the convenience of a light bulb.

---

ottlite.com

(800) 842-8848
Monday – Friday 8:30 a.m. – 5 p.m. EST
(excluding major holidays)

Many other companies now also offer full-spectrum light bulbs. These companies, and the lights they carry, can be found by typing **"full-spectrum light bulbs"** in the address bar of your browser.

Books on full-spectrum lighting and sunlight that may interest you:

- *Health and Light-The Extraordinary Study that Shows How Light Affects Your Health and Emotional Well-Being*, by John N. Ott

- *Light, Radiation, and You-How to Stay Healthy*, by John N. Ott

- *The Healing Sun: Sunlight and Health in the 21st Century*, by Richard Hobday

- *Sunlight Could Save Your Life*, by Dr. Zane Klime

- *Light: Medicine of the Future: How We Can Use It to Heal Ourselves Now*, by Jacob Lieberman

ESSENTIALS FOR THE CAREGIVER

An action plan is necessary. The topics below cover the basic survival needs in any caregiver's life. It is important that these areas become priorities. When they do, they will make life a whole lot easier and a lot less stressful. Consult with your physician or other licensed healthcare professional regarding any potential food allergies you may have to the foods mentioned in this section.

Eating

Eating properly does not often rank high on a caregiver's priority list.

This is especially true if you are a full-time caregiver, and the demands of everyday living become an overwhelming and daunting task.

Also remember that skipping meals may easily cause your blood sugar levels to fluctuate. This fluctuation may also create feelings of fatigue, depression, and other physical and emotional changes. Perhaps many of you have already experienced this.

Time is a premium commodity for most caregivers. The less time you spend in the kitchen, the more you will want to take a meal break. This also applies to making meals for your loved one.

So what's the solution?

I found that efficient small appliances that make food preparation *quick and easy* will become your best friends. With your new friends ready for action, you will now be able to eat a nutritious meal in minutes, with minimal cleanup and time to spare.

Note from Camille:

These are the products I used or discovered while caregiving. If you are satisfied with the appliances you are currently using, by all means continue to use them. I found the following small appliances a breeze to work with, with minimal time and effort in the kitchen. The last three items listed were not available during my caregiving days (excluding the juicer), and are included here because they are fast, efficient, and can produce delicious meals in 10 minutes or less. I use them all now, and can vouch for their ease and simplicity.

Electric Egg Cooker

- Make poached, soft, and hard-boiled eggs in a snap
- Place eggs in cooker with a predetermined amount of water, and presto, the eggs are cooked to perfection every time

- The cooker chirps when done

- No babysitting required

- If you have never used an egg cooker before, I think once you use it, you will wonder how you ever survived without it!

- Many brands to choose from

- May be purchased from a variety of locations, including online

- Price range: $15 to $30

Panini Maker

- Fast and easy to use

- Grill plates on panini makers are generally hotter than other similar appliances

- Has floating hinged grill plate on top, which remains parallel to the bottom grill plate

  - This allows for even browning or searing of all food or sandwiches, no matter what thickness

- Easy clean up

- Many brands to choose from

- May be purchased from many retail stores or online

- Price range: $45 to $69 (average)

Ninja®Express Chopper

- Mini food chopper

- Pulsed or full chop

- Small container makes it easy to use and control

- Useful in making quick meals, salsa, dressings, sauces, and spreads

- Easy to clean

- Excellent for chopping celery, onions, tomatoes, spices, herbs, nuts, chocolate, and just about anything else you can think of—quickly and easily

- Easy to prepare chicken salad or egg salad in seconds

  - Just toss all ingredients in the container, pulse a few seconds, add a little mayo, and voila!

- ▪ Remember, you already cooked the hard boiled eggs in the electric egg cooker without devoting any conscious attention to cooking them...

   AND

- ▪ You may have also cooked the chicken breasts in the Air Fryer (see below), so they too, are ready for you!

- ▪ Hmmm... You just might want to make both salads at the same time, saving even more time later... ☺

- ● Available from retail outlets or online

- ● Price: $25 or less

This little gadget saved the day many times when I needed a quick meal in minutes.
You will be amazed how often you will use this device. It is small enough to be convenient, and convenient enough to use often.

Rice Cooker:

- ● Several styles are available

- ● Those easiest to operate have a 'one button' control

- ● First it cooks the food, then shuts off automatically to keep the food warm until you are ready to eat

   - ▪ The food is always ready whenever you are, without fear of burning or scorching

- ● Again, no babysitting required

- ● Perfect rice every time

- ● Cooks more than just rice:

   - ▪ Soups

   - ▪ Casseroles

   - ▪ Macaroni and cheese

   - ▪ And much more...

- ● Easy to operate

- ● Various brands available

- ● Various sizes available: 3, 5, 7, 8, & 10 cups being the most popular

- ● Price: $25 on up, depending on size and brand chosen

Rice cooker cookbook suggestions (for other recipes besides rice):

- *Mini Rice Cooker Cookbook*, by Lynda Balslev
- *The Ultimate Rice Cooker Cookbook*, by Beth Hensperger & Julie Kaufmann

There are many other cookbooks available using rice cookers for recipes other than rice. Investigate and experiment and create your own unique dishes.

NutriBullet®Rx or Nutri Ninja®Auto iQ™ Pro Complete

- Super easy to use
- Ideal smoothie maker
- Includes several shatterproof tumblers (various sizes)
  - Tumblers also serve as the mixing container
  - Tumblers also serve as 'on-the-go' drinking container
- Great for quick liquid meal
- Totally emulsifies fruits, veggies, nuts, and seeds for complete consumption of all nutrients, including the pulp
- Self-contained and easy cleanup
- Small footprint on countertop
- Available from most retail stores and online
- Price: $125 to $200 depending on make and model

Air Fryer

- Gaining rapid popularity
- Footprint the size of a bread maker (although larger models are now available)
- Uses only air and heat to cook
- Meals in literally minutes
- Easy clean up
- Foods taste like they were either fried or seared on a grill
- Great for veggies (tasty snacks in minutes—French fries taste like they were deep fried!)
- Great for fish and poultry

- Will find yourself using this appliance almost every day

- Available in retail outlets or online

- Price: $100 to $500 depending on make and model chosen

Stone Wave™ Ceramic Microwave Cooker

- Makes omelets in 2 to 3 minutes, depending how many 'goodies' you add to the omelet

  - **Example**: Scramble 2 eggs directly in the ceramic container; add anything you wish like tomato, onion, green peppers, mushrooms; top with shredded cheese; pop in microwave for 2 to 3 minutes, and you have a perfect omelet every time!

- Makes other quick little meals in 5 to 10 minutes (recipes included)

- Shape is similar to an old fashioned small bean pot with open chimney lid

- One of the best little gifts I ever received, and use it often

- Price: $20 or less

Juicers

- Takes a little bit more time to prepare juice, but well worth the effort

- Including here, because juicing is one of the fastest and easiest ways to absorb nutrients directly in the cells without having to go through hours of digestion

- Different from the NutriBullet®Rx or NutriNinja®, as the pulp is extracted from the juice

- Makes delicious nutritious drinks for pennies, especially if you grow your own fruits and vegetables

- Price: $100 to $200 (average)

It is often difficult, if not impractical, to eat the recommended quantity of fruits and vegetables every day. Therefore, juicing and smoothies are a great way to consume raw fruits and vegetables in the quantities that are most beneficial. It is also a way to consume them in their natural, raw state.

There are many excellent juicers on the market to choose from...
It is a personal preference as to what qualities you are looking for.

Note from Camille:

I personally own the JackLaLanne™ juicer for many reasons; including the fact it has a wider opening for inserting the food, and is easy to clean. The wider opening eliminates much of the prep time by not having to cut the food to fit the opening. Whole apples and pears easily fit into the opening without having to cut them. The Breville® Juice Fountain™ Plus is also a good choice—with a wide opening, dual speed control for hard and softer fruits and veggies, and also easy to clean. Price: Under $150.

Money Saving Tip:

If there is a **Bed Bath and Beyond** store in your area, you may want to use their **$5 off** and **20% off** coupons. If you subscribe to their mailing list, they send these coupons regularly, and the coupons never expire. The coupons may be applied to anything they sell, so you can easily save a tremendous amount of money this way.

Sleeping

Although sleep is vitally important, many caregivers are overextending themselves to the point of exhaustion. When this occurs, physical and emotional changes also begin to take place.

If you have *already* reached this point, I suggest you take a one-to two-week vacation. Give yourself permission to do this, and please refer to **Out-of-Home Respite Care (page 156).**

Obtaining restful, restorative sleep is often challenging. This is even more intensified in the elderly.

In order to heal and rejuvenate the body, a person must enter the stage of deep sleep known as the "delta" level. This is the level where restorative healing takes place.

Many seniors, menopausal, and perimenopausal women, are not able to reach this delta level due to medications, pain, sleep apnea, hormonal changes, and other physical conditions. If you are stressed, overwhelmed, worried, or pre-occupied with other emotions that clutter the mind with endless chatter, you may not be able to reach this delta level, no matter what your age.

The information below will help you better understand why proper rest is so important.

The Five Stages of sleep are:

- Stage 1—transition between awake and asleep
- Stage 2—THETA sleep, baseline sleep
- Stage 3 & 4—DELTA sleep
- Stage 5—REM sleep (Rapid Eye Movement sleep, where dreaming occurs)

Essentials of 'delta' level sleep:

- Necessary for healing and rejuvenation of the body
- Necessary for proper brain function
- Lack of delta sleep may cause behavior that mimics signs of dementia or Alzheimer's such as:
  - Forgetfulness
  - Poor decision making
  - Brain fog
  - Confusion
  - Delayed response time
  - Drunk-like stupor

Preparing the body for sleep

It is essential to prepare the body for sleep. This is especially true if a person has difficulty sleeping in general, or for any of the reasons mentioned above.

Some suggestions of natural over-the-counter products which may be helpful in obtaining the deeper delta levels of sleep are listed below. These over-the-counter products are *not* sleeping pills. Thus, they do not have the side effects that many prescription sleeping pills exhibit.

*** These examples are included for informational purposes only.***

As always, consult with your physician or healthcare professional first, before adding any vitamins, herbs, or other over-the-counter products to your regimen.
If you and your physician decide these over-the-counter products are worth investigating, try one product at a time, to see which product works best for you.

1. **Over-the-counter products that aid in sleeping**:
   - **Melatonin**
     - Body manufactures this natural hormone
     - Turns off with daylight, turns on with darkness
     - Important for the body to differentiate between day and night
     - Responsible for 'jet lag' if not in proper supply

- o Decreases as we age
- o May be taken 30 minutes prior to bedtime to help signal the body to sleep

- **L-Tryptophan**
  - o An essential amino acid
  - o Converts serotonin to melatonin in the body (see 'melatonin' above)
  - o Found in sardines, tuna, milk, and turkey (most commonly)—this is why you often feel sleepy after consuming these foods

It is not advisable to eat a large meal before attempting to sleep, even if the meal contains tryptophan. A large meal should be consumed at least three to four hours before bedtime. If you are hungry and must eat something, eat a small amount, and only foods that are easy to digest. Otherwise, the body spends the night digesting instead of resting, repairing, and restoring itself, and delta level sleep is not obtained. You often wake up tired when a heavy meal is consumed prior to sleeping the night before.

- **Alteril™**
  - o Natural over-the-counter product
  - o Available online or retail stores
  - o Contains L-tryptophan, passionflower, valerian root, melatonin, chamomile
  - o Allows easy drifting into delta and REM sleep
  - o Wake up refreshed

2. **Helpful tips to obtain quality sleep**:

- **Pillows**
  - o A proper pillow is an important consideration in obtaining good sleep quality
  - o If you awaken with a stiff neck, headache, numbness, or painful shoulders—part of the problem may be the pillow you are sleeping on
  - o Having the cervical portion of the neck supported is also important

If you currently do not have a pillow that offers the support needed, you may want to simply roll up a hand towel (rolled into a cylinder), and place it under your neck. This will offer temporary support to the cervical region, until you are able to purchase a pillow that will help accomplish this.

There are a variety of excellent pillow companies available in the marketplace, and you may need to experiment to find a pillow that best fits your body size, head, and neck. You can then determine which pillow(s) simply feels the most comfortable and provides the most support for restful sleep.

- **Positioning the Body**

  Sleep on your side or on your back (with knees bent), and avoid sleeping on your stomach.

  Stomach sleeping distorts the cervical spine, and is a contributing factor to the pain and stiffness you may experience both during sleep, and upon awakening.

- **Eating before bed**

  Avoid eating a large heavy meal directly before bedtime.

  Avoid caffeine (including coffee and chocolate), sugary or high-carbohydrate foods (including ice cream, cookies, cake, and candy), spicy or fatty foods, and alcohol.

  All of the above may keep you awake, and prevent you from sleeping soundly.

  Meals containing large amounts of protein (like meat), will take longer to digest than other food(s), and you will spend most of the night digesting instead of resting, healing, and restoring your body. You will often wake up tired the next day.

- **No television, laptops, or cell phones in the bedroom**

  The glow from the above devices emits a 'blue' light if left on through the night.

  'Blue' light from electronic devices prevents the pineal gland from producing melatonin, the hormone which regulates day and night, or sleep / wake cycles.

  Decreased melatonin will prevent delta and REM sleep levels from occurring.

- **Decrease room light exposure when attempting to sleep**

  Light (any light) interferes with the body's melatonin production—which is active during sleep and darkness, and upsets the body's circadian rhythm.

  The room should be as dark as possible for restful, restorative sleep.

- **Eye masks**

  An eye mask is very beneficial in helping to increase sleep quality.

  The mask further blocks out light, and delta and REM sleep levels are attained more quickly.

  Try using an eye mask for a few days. I think you will notice a difference in feeling more rested and refreshed upon awaking.

- **Napping**

  It is often difficult to obtain a full night sleep, especially while caregiving.

  A good time to nap is when your loved one is also napping.

  Ideal nap time is 10 to 20 minutes—more than that may leave you groggy.

  One 10- to 20-minute nap is often all you need to help restore energy and vitality.

  Naps can...
  - Reduce drowsiness and fatigue
  - Increase alertness
  - Improve cognitive performance
  - Sharpen motor skills
  - Improve mood

  Nap tips:
  - Set timer for no more than 20 minutes
  - Lie down on a comfortable surface
  - Put on eye mask to eliminate light (black masks will block more light)
    - Total darkness induces faster sleep
  - Wake up refreshed!

- **Aromatherapy**

  Lavender and lavender oil have been used for centuries to help induce sleep with its calming qualities (make sure it is pure lavender and not a synthetic imitation).

  Pure lavender oil and dried lavender flowers may be purchased from many sources:
  - Online
  - Health food stores or other retail stores

  You may also purchase a diffuser to help distribute the fragrance in the room.

  Spray a diluted version of the oil on bed linen and pillows, providing even more relaxation. You may dilute the oil with simple tap water. Shake the sprayer bottle before use. The dried flowers may be placed in small organza bags and made into sachets.

- **Music that's helpful for sleep**
  - *Solaris Universalis* and *Atlantis Angelis (Volume I),* by Patrick Bernard
    - The music and sounds on both albums are very specific for healing the body
    - Maybe purchased on Patrick's website: **patrickbernard.com**
      - Able to hear sound-bites of all songs on his website before purchasing
      - Many new albums are now also available

There has been a name change from Patrick Bernhardt to Patrick Bernard. Some of his music still has his former name on the albums. The content is the same.

Note from Camille*:*

I used both albums above when caring for my mother. They were played daily throughout the night, with very noticeable positive effects.

- *Delta Sleep System: Fall Asleep, Stay Asleep, Wake Up Rejuvenated*, by Dr. Jeffrey Thompson
  - Clinically proven audio technology
  - Available through: **www.soundstrue.com**

All the music suggestions above may be played throughout the night, and will assist in obtaining a deeper quality of healing sleep while they are being played.

- Other Suggestions:
  - Ask a family member or friend to sit with your loved one while you sleep
  - Take advantage of some **FREE** respite options provided in this Resource Guide

Respite Care

If you are a 24 / 7 caregiver, frequent breaks are absolutely necessary.

At the very least, take 5 to 10 minutes every few hours to walk outside, meditate, stretch, shake your body out, or simply close your eyes.

Besides family and friends, please refer to your **local AREA AGENCY on AGING (page 26)**, **RESPITE CARE (page 156)**, and **MISCELLANEOUS ORGANIZATIONS (page 190)** sections of this Resource Guide. There are organizations in the MO section which provide respite care relief for **FREE** or **low-cost**. Scroll through the list(s), then call and inquire.

The hours allocated for respite through different government programs may vary based on multiple factors, including need.

Speak to the social worker or nurse that has been assigned to the case. Be honest with that person. If you are exhausted, let the person know. That's what the programs are there for!

Utilize the resources above, and don't forget to ask for help!

Suggestions:

- Obtain scheduled respite care at least once a week
- Leave the house during the time respite care is provided, unless you are so exhausted you simply need that time to sleep
- Ask family members or friends to relieve you often
- *Be firm in your asking!*

Stress Reduction

- Overall well-being is improved when stress levels are reduced
- Caring for a loved one with continuous needs is obviously stressful
- Depression and anxiety may likely occur if precautionary measures are not taken
- The suggestions below will help you obtain a more calming and positive internal and external environment
  - Some of these suggestions do not require any active participation on your part, yet may make an incredible, immediate, observable difference in your life

Helpful Suggestions to Decrease Stress:

- Play soothing music

- Aromatherapy

- Meditation and Prayer

- Art therapy

- Fish tanks and pets

- Chiropractic

- Massage

- Acupuncture and Acupressure

- Energy Balancing

- Therapeutic mineral baths

- Spa

- Whirlpool

- Yoga

- T'ai Chi

- Socializing with friends

- Exercise

  - Reduces stress

  - Increases energy and positive outlook

  - Increases endorphins

  - Walking even short distances for 5 to 10 minutes will help

  - Rebounding on a mini-trampoline

    o Fun and easy to do

    o Urban Rebounder™ (brand of mini-trampoline)—may purchase online

- Sunshine and fresh air

  - Increases Vitamin D levels

  - Very healing and increases better mood

  - Spend at least 20 to 30 minutes outside (even in the winter)

- Adopt a pet

Personal note from Camille:

Shortly before my mother's death, I adopted my first rescued pet (a Doberman I named Grace), from a local Doberman Rescue. Even though I have had pets all my life, I was told by many that once you adopt, you will always adopt, because there is unique and special bond that develops between the rescued pet and new owner. I found this to be absolutely true.

Grace proved to be a devoted and loving companion, and was the happiest dog I ever owned. She just seemed happy to be alive, as if she somehow knew I saved her life. After my mother's death, it was Grace who then saved me. She provided the comfort, solace, and peace I needed when my heart was aching and my soul was grieving.

I share this with you, because pets like Grace offer such unconditional love without asking for anything in return. There are many animals like Grace available through various rescue services and animal shelters. Consider adopting, as these animals will prove to be faithful and loyal companions that just seem to know when you're feeling a little down or troubled.

They will provide comfort when you need it most, a listening ear when you need to talk, and a source of unconditional love when you may not be very lovable.

Think about it... Your new friend is waiting for you!

Video Stories

The following websites are *excellent* for viewing a variety of situations and documentaries regarding the various aspects of caregiving.

Just seeing and witnessing others in your same situation, may be helpful to you, and you may also gain some helpful tips.

videocaregiving.org
- Provides visual education for family caregivers of loved ones with Alzheimer's, strokes, or other physical disabilities

besmartbewell.com

To the Family and Friends of a Caregiver

Stop by and visit as often as possible. To the caregiver, it is always nice to see a friendly face, even if you can only spare 10 to 15 minutes.

Your help is needed even if the caregiver does not ask you. In fact, caregivers are often so caught up and overwhelmed in their daily duties, they may not know what help is even needed.

While doing research for this book, I asked random caregivers what they would ask for most, if someone was kind enough to help them out.

The results were unanimous!

The top two desires were REST and / or TIME AWAY and a GOOD NUTRITIOUS MEAL!

REST and FOOD are two basic necessities of life, and so vital for caregiver survival.

Help a caregiver out in any way possible, especially in the two areas mentioned above. Be assured that *any* help you offer them will be greatly appreciated.

Suggestions to help a caregiver you may know:

At the top of their wish list, caregivers would love a little time off. Offer to sit with their loved one, if only for a few hours!

1. Bring a meal.
2. Take the caregiver to dinner.
3. Sit with the bedridden person for a few hours so the caregiver can rest.
4. Mow the lawn.
5. Take out the garbage.
6. Go shopping for food or items that are needed.
7. Wash the dishes.
8. Check the batteries on the smoke detectors.
9. Change the furnace filter.
10. Look outside to see if there is some exterior maintenance that needs to be done.
11. Call them, even if you cannot visit. This way you let them know you are thinking about them and they haven't been forgotten.

RESOURCE BOOKS regarding the emotional aspects of caregiving:

- *The Emotional Survival Guide for Caregivers: Looking After Yourself and Your Family While Helping an Aging Parent*, Barry J. Jacobs PsyD

- *Mainstay: For the Well Spouse of the Chronically Ill*, Maggie Strong

- *Chicken Soup for the Caregiver's Soul*, Jack Canfield, Mark Victor Hansen, LeAnn Thieman, LPN

These are only a few of the books available to assist you.
There are many more to choose from depending on your own specific needs.

CHECKLISTSFOR EMOTIONAL CARE

Note: *Author grants permission for you to make copies of this checklist for your future needs and as your information changes.*

ACTION PLAN FOR EATING

Scheduled time for eating	
Products that could be helpful	
Asking for help from family / friends to help cook / bring meals over	

ACTION PLAN FOR SLEEPING

Scheduled time for sleeping	
Products that could be helpful	
Asking for help from family / friends to schedule naps / rest periods	

ACTION PLAN FOR RESPITE CARE

Program name	
Phone	
Contact person	
Scheduled time for weekly respite care	
Scheduled time for vacation respite care	

ACTION PLAN FOR STRESS REDUCTION

Planned activity	
Time of day for activity	
Scheduled amount of time	

Begin with SOMETHING—even if it's only for five minutes!

LEGISLATION

"The ultimate rulers of our democracy are not a president and senators and congressmen and government officials—but the voters of this country."

—Franklin D. Roosevelt

LEGISLATION

There are always bills in congress that will directly or indirectly impact the government programs available for caregivers.

While it may be impossible to know every bill that is being considered, written, or debated—it is wise to follow the most current news and voice your opinions to your elected officials.

It is vitally important that government officials become even more aware of what help and assistance is needed in caregiver families.

We all must encourage our elected officials to provide bills that will assist the caregiver in more ways than are currently being offered.

> To find your representatives in Congress, please visit:
>
> **congress.org**

- From the home page, you will be able to contact your local lawmakers

  - Enter your **zip code** and **email** address in the box

    - Will provide links to send emails to **your** members of Congress using pre-addressed forms

  - Write to your congressmen (both senators and representatives) with your concerns—**every voice counts!**

It is so important for family caregivers to contact their respective members of Congress. Tell them you are a family caregiver, and what changes you would like to see happen to make your life easier. Remember, every voice counts, and one voice speaks very loudly for many in the silent majority!

- Family Caregivers in the U.S. (2017) provided approximately **$470 billion** dollars in unpaid care, support, and other services by providing **FREE** 'In-Home' care **(34 billion hours)**—rather than putting their qualified Medicaid loved one in a Nursing Home

- Cost of annual basic Nursing Home Care hovers around $80,000+ per year

- Statistics show that loved ones do better in their own homes

- By contacting your representatives and senators and letting them know how you feel, they will be better equipped to initiate various bills to help, educate, and financially compensate hard working family members like yourself

  - These family members must often quit their jobs (thus losing even more money, benefits, and services) to help care for their loved ones

The **Paid Family Leave Act (H.R. 1439/S.786)** was introduced by Rep. Rosa DeLauro (D-CT) & Sen. Kirsten Gillibrand (D-NY). This bill would ensure that a person would be entitled to 12 weeks of paid compensation—at a percentage of their weekly wage—in order to care for themselves or a loved one. So far, this bill has NOT been passed.

Please contact your government officials, and ask them to pass this bill into law.

Some states DO have a Paid Family Leave program in place (California, New Jersey, Rhode Island, Washington, DC, New York, and Massachusetts). Eligibility to qualify for these programs must be met, as with all programs.

Social Security Benefits

The last cost-of-living adjustment (COLA) occurred in January 2021 (1.3%).

There were no cost-of-living adjustments in 2010, 2011 and 2016, which are the only three years with no increase since the COLA was put into effect in 1975.

Although Social Security is a volatile topic in Congress, those who are already obtaining benefits should continue to receive them. Only time will tell...

Filial Laws

Filial laws are important laws you may not be aware of. These laws may affect you, whether you know about them or not.

Many states have laws which could make an adult child responsible for the financing of their parents' care.

These laws are referred to as "filial support (responsibility) laws."

The laws vary from state to state, and could include criminal penalties.

Most cases do not go to court. However, even though most cases do not—several have—leaving the family member responsible for the bills. It's important to be aware of this law if you live in a state with filial laws still on the books.

You may want to write your state representatives to have the law removed in your state.

> For a list of states with Filial Laws, please visit:
>
> **https://www.agingcare.com/articles/filial-responsibility-and-medicaid-197746.htm**

RESOURCES CONSULTED

"Benefits & Eligibility for the Aid & Attendance, Housebound & Basic Pensions for Veterans & Surviving Spouses." American Council on Aging. Updated October 10, 2019. https://www.medicaidplanningassistance.org/va-pension-aid-and-attendance/.

"Blue Light Disturbs Sleep, Especially in Teen-Agers," Meerl Kim, *The Washington Post*, Sept. 1, 2014.

Cannuscio, C.C., C. Jones, I. Kawachi, G.A. Colditz, L. Berkman and E. Rimm, "Reverberation of Family Illness: A longitudinal assessment of informal caregiver and mental health status in the nurses' health study." *American Journal of Public Health* 92:305-1311, 2002.

"Cost of Care Survey 2019," Genworth. Nov. 21, 2019. https://www.genworth.com/aging-and-you/finances/cost-of-care.html.

"Cost-of-Living Adjustment (COLA) Information for 2021." Social Security. https://www.ssa.gov/cola/

Drs. Janice-Kiecolt Glaser and Ronald Glaser, "Chronic stress and age-related increases in the proinflammatory cytokine IL-6." *Proceedings of the National Academy of Sciences*, June 30, 2003.

Elissa S. Epel, Dept of Psychiatry, University of California, SF, et al, *Proceedings of the National Academy of Sciences*, Dec 7, 2004, Vol. 101, No. 49.

"The Family and Medical Insurance Leave Act," (Fact Sheet), *National Partnership for Females & Families*, March 2015.

Health and Human Services, "Informal Caregiving: Compassion in Action. Washington, DC: Department of Health and Human Services." Based on data from the National Survey of Families and Households (NSFH), 1998 and the National Family Caregivers Association, Random Sample Survey of Family Caregivers, Summer 2000, Unpublished and National Alliance for Caregiving and AARP, Caregiving in the U.S., 2004.

Heiser, K. Gabriel. "Filial Responsibility Laws and Medicaid." Aging Care. Updated June 20, 2019. https://www.agingcare.com/articles/filial-responsibility-and-medicaid-197746.htm.

"How to compare Medigap policies." Medicare. Accessed December 31, 2019. https://www.medicare.gov/supplements-other-insurance/how-to-compare-medigap-policies.

"Lavender-The Sweet Smell of Sleep," Sara Altshul, *Prevention*, November 3, 2011.

Lewis, Christina L. "FAQs for businesses on the Massachusetts Paid Family Leave Law." *Boston Business Journal*, September 13, 2019. https://www.bizjournals.com/boston/news/2019/09/13/faqs-for-businesses-on-the-massachusetts-paid.html.

"Millions Face Shrinking Social Security Payments," Stephen Ohlemacher, Associated Press Writer, Aug 23, 2009.

Nicholas D. Christakis, Professor, Healthcare Policy, Harvard Medical School, Boston and Suzanne Salamon, M.D., Associate Chief, Geriatric Psychiatry, Beth Israel Deaconess Hospital, Boston, *New England Journal of Medicine*, Feb. 16, 2006.

"No Cost of Living Increase in 2016," Jeffry Bartash, *Market Watch*, October 15, 2015.

Norris, Louise. "How are Medicare Benefits Changing for 2020." Medicare Resources. Dec. 13, 2019. https://www.medicareresources.org/faqs/what-kind-of-medicare-benefit-changes-can-i-expect-this-year/.

Schulz, R. and Beach, S. R., "Caregiving as a Risk Factor for Mortality: The Caregiver Health Effects Study." *Journal of the American Medical Association*, Vol. 282, No. 23, December 15, 1999.

"Sleep Away the Pounds, Optimize Your Sleep and Reset Your Metabolism for Maximum Weight Loss," by Cherie Calbom, MS, with John Calbom, MA, January 2007.

"Six Conditions That Feel Like Clinical Depression But Aren't," Therese Borchard, *Everyday Health*, June 5, 2014.

"Sleepy After a Big Meal? Here's Why," *Huffington Post*, November 22, 2012.

"Social Security: The Lump-Sum Death Benefit," Noah P. Myerson, Analyst in Income Security, *Congressional Research Service,* July 15, 2014.

"State Paid Family Leave Insurance Laws" chart*, National Partnership for Women and Families,* February 2015.

"Taking Care of Our Own," by Lauren Sandler, *New Republic*, March 18, 2015.

"The Positive Health Benefits of Negative Ions," Jim English, *Nutrition Review*, April 22, 2013.

"Valuating the Invaluable: 2015 Update," by Susan C. Reinhard, Lynn Friss Feinberg, Rita Choula, and Ari Houser, Insight on the Issues, July 2015, AARP Public Policy Institute.

"What Paid Family Leave Looks Like In The Three States That Offer It," by Niraj Chokskl, *The Washington Post*, June 14, 2014.

"What You Need to Know About NJ Paid Family Leave Law," by Stark and Stark, *Employment*, March 26, 2009.

"Who Will Pay for Mom's or Dad's Nursing Home Bill? Filial Support Laws And Long-Term Care," Northwestern Mutual Voice Team, *Forbes*, Feb. 3, 2014.

PROFESSIONAL RESOURCES CONSULTED

Hector Bultynck, C.P.A.
David Bultynck, C.P.A.
Bultynck & Co, PC
15985 Canal Road
Clinton Township, MI 48038
(586) 286-7300

John D. Cadieux
Attorney at Law
1700 W. Hamlin Road Suite #100
Rochester Hills, MI 48309
(248) 652-3608

Steve Sheldon, D.C., F.I.C.P.A
32 S. Squirrel Road
Auburn Hills, MI 48326
(248) 289-6870

QUICK REFERENCE GUIDE

BOOKS

The Emotional Survival Guide for Caregivers: Looking After Yourself and Your Family While Helping an Aging Parent, by Barry J. Jacobs PsyD, 1997-2009

Mainstay: For the Well Spouse of the Chronically Ill, by Maggie Strong

Chicken Soup for the Caregiver's Soul, by Jack Canfield, Mark Victor Hansen, LeAnn Thieman, LPN

Health and Light-The Extraordinary Study that Shows How Light Affects Your Health and Emotional Well-Being, by John N. Ott

Light, Radiation, and You: How to Stay Healthy, by John N. Ott

The Healing Sun: Sunlight and Health in the 21st Century, by Richard Hobday

Sunlight Could Save Your Life, by Dr. Zane Klime

Mini Rice Cooker Cookbook, by Lynda Balslev

The Ultimate Rice Cooker Cookbook, by Beth Hensperger & Julie Kaufmann

CDs and MP3s

Solaris Universalis & Atlantis Angelis (Vol. I), by Patrick Bernard

- Available through Patrick's website: **www.patrickbernard.com**
- May listen to sound bites from all albums before you buy

Healing Mind System, by Dr. Jeffrey Thompson

Delta Sleep System: Fall Asleep, Stay Asleep, Wake Up Rejuvenated, by Dr. Jeffrey Thompson

- Available through: soundstrue.com

ADDITIONAL COPIES OF THIS RESOURCE GUIDE may be purchased on Amazon.com.

To book Dr. Superson as your next speaker and / or for bulk orders, you may email her directly at Camille@DrCamilleSuperson.com or call toll free **(844) 780-9962**.

REQUEST FOR REVIEWS

Thank you in advance for taking a moment to post a review for *Essential Resource Guide for Caregivers* on Amazon.com.

Taking that extra step is important… as your review may be extremely instrumental in helping others decide how this book can directly help them, their friends, and their families.

If you enjoyed reading *Essential Resource Guide for Caregivers,* I deeply appreciate your efforts in helping others to discover and enjoy the book as well.

Being a caregiver myself for many years in the past, I know I was always searching for viable resources to help both me and my family.

You can help spread the word in a variety of ways:

LEND IT: The digital version of this book is lending enabled, so please feel free to share it with a friend.

RECOMMEND IT: Please help other readers discover this book by recommending it to various readers groups, caregiver groups, Goodreads, on your Facebook page, Pinterest, Twitter, Instagram, discussion boards, various social media pages, and by sharing the information directly through word of mouth.

REVIEW IT: Please share with others why you liked this book by reviewing it on the site where you purchased it, on your favorite book site, on your own blog and / or website, on Facebook, Pinterest, Twitter, Instagram, and LinkedIn.

EMAIL ME: I would love to hear from you! I would especially love to hear how this Resource Guide personally and specifically provided the information and resources you needed to help make your life a little easier and more stress-free!

Camille@DrCamilleSuperson.com

Thank you so much!

With sincere gratitude…

Camille

ACKNOWLEDGEMENTS

During the course of my life, there have been some very special people who appeared like Guardian Angels, at just the right time when I needed them most. They were like the North Star, directing me through the darkness and into the light.

At critical times, when both parents were very ill, when the future seemed bleak, and when it took everything I had to keep from entering emotional places that were disempowering—my Guardian Angels began to appear.

The word *HOPE* now had a new meaning to me, and the gratitude I feel for the following individuals can never be fully expressed in words alone.

I extend a special thank you to all of them for their generosity, time, love, and guidance during a most difficult time.

To Terese Gostomski: You always seemed to appear when I needed you most. You often offered help without being asked, and I cannot tell you what it meant for you to be there and care for Mom when I needed to sleep, relax, move from Chicago to Michigan, and tie up loose ends. You often treated me to dinner, never knowing how much I needed that time to clear my mind. Without you, I would have not discovered the Waiver Program and all the assistance that program provided. I will miss you.

To Flo Brana: You were there for me in areas I never anticipated. You assisted in directing me to top notch professionals to help deal with all the unexpected and endless surprises I encountered along the way. You were there to provide support by checking in periodically to make sure we were okay, and letting me know that you were always just a phone call away. Thank you for taking me to dinner when you visited, and always being a friend to Mom and me—just as you had been to Dad. May you continue your friendship with Dad in Heaven.

To Dennis Hartwick: You always found time to help. Thank you for cutting the grass, removing downed trees from the yard, making minor repairs around the house, and for helping with Dad when he was hospitalized and unable to feed or shave himself. I knew I could always count on you, and you became a rock I could lean on. I will always remember and cherish your kindnesses.

To John Cadieux: You are one of the best lawyers I know. You were, and are, always there for me through all the legal issues I ever had to deal with. You became like family to me and I appreciate you more than you will ever know. Thank you for continuing to always be there, and always being just a phone call away.

To Hector Bultynck: You provided your accounting expertise during many trying times, especially at the beginning. Thank you for helping to make sense out of the endless piles of paper I 'inherited.' I will always be grateful for your help and guidance. You became a trusted friend and I will miss you terribly. Your time on this earth was far too short.

To Dr. Vahagn Agbabian: You provided such excellent medical care to Mom. You took time to actually *listen*, and your concern for her was always a top priority. I especially want to thank you for the respect you always showed her, and the respect and trust in my abilities to use and incorporate the knowledge I had acquired. Most of all, I appreciated your constant support during many difficult times. I respect and honor you in more ways than you can ever imagine. I will always feel blessed that you were our doctor. Like so many others, I will miss your gentle ways and your selfless compassion for others. I know Mom is very happy to see you!

To Pastor David Boone: You were a true friend to our family for decades. You had the ability to allow Dad to feel safe in your presence and share the heavy burdens in his heart. Your years of kindness to our family will not be forgotten. I am so grateful you were there when I needed someone to turn to and talk with.

To Dr. Steve Sheldon: Thank you for always doing your best to keep my body pain-free and mobile through all the years of heavy lifting that was required in caring for a bedbound person. You helped me so many times when I could barely move. I don't know what I would have done without you. You're the best!

To Mary DeAmparo: Thank you for always being there for me, for being my 'long-distance' secretary after my sudden move to Michigan to care for my parents, for helping me pack up my house, and your help in fulfilling my father's wishes. I hold you close to my heart, and you will always be "family" to me—cherished deeply, and loved unconditionally.

To Dr. Arthur Parrott: Some of the most important gifts you gave me were your support and love during a very stressful time. Thank you for your active participation in helping to fulfill my father's wishes. It meant so much, and I will always cherish your kindness and friendship.

To Greg & Linda Sobotka: You went beyond the call of duty as neighbors. You were always there to help, no matter what! I am thankful and grateful to both of you for going out of your way to take care of my home and making it looked 'lived in' when I couldn't be there to do it myself. Your kindnesses will never be forgotten. Thank you so much!

To Ann Videan: How can I ever thank you enough? Without you, this book would not have taken physical form, and your integrity, loyalty, and dedication to making this book a reality goes beyond any thank you I can ever give you. You are a special angel to me, and I feel richly blessed and humbly grateful. Thank you from the bottom of my heart!

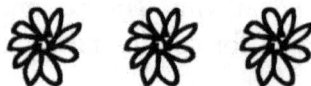

❋ ❋ ❋

BEYOND THE BOOK

Dr. Camille Superson provides consulting and training to corporations, associations, organizations, and small businesses on how to improve bottom-line profits.

Through educating caregiver team members on how to find the resources they need, the reduced stress and elimination of wasted time looking for information helps valued team members become more focused on their work.

Everyone WINS! And this valuable information will bring a new joy and peace both at home and in the workplace. This becomes even more important with so many individuals now working from home.

Dr. Superson can also customize a special presentation for your audience and team members.

For more information, email Dr. Superson at Camille@DrCamilleSuperson.com

For your **FREE** gift, please go to StressFreeCaregiver.com and download your personal copy of the *Quick Start Guide for Caregivers.*

ABOUT THE AUTHOR

Dr. Camille Superson is the author of the ESSENTIAL RESOURCE GUIDE FOR CAREGIVERS: Save TIME… Save MONEY… Save Your SANITY!!!

After a fulfilling career as a pharmacist, chiropractor, and owner of one of the first comprehensive holistic clinics in metro Chicago, life was abruptly altered when she became a 24/7 full-time caregiver to two bedbound parents—which spanned over a decade.

Challenges were many, and finding the needed help and resources to care for both parents was overwhelming and stressful.

These struggles propelled her to become a caregiver advocate and author—providing caregivers and their families with valuable access to many of the **FREE** or **nearly-free** hard-to-find resources available.

Teaching, speaking, and sharing this information with groups, organizations, and individuals became a calling that would not let go.

Showing people how to avoid the stresses and pitfalls associated with caring for a loved one—while still living a relatively normal life—became a mission.

She brings hope, simplicity, and order to a potentially complex situation, and has the ability to help others find joy in an often lonely, isolated, yet incredible journey. This is her gift!

She is a frequent guest on a variety of radio shows throughout the United States and Canada, where she shares this crucial information with their audiences.

Visit StressFreeCaregiver.com for your FREE gift—the *Quick Start Guide for Caregivers* or call

(844) 780-9962 for more information. For media interviews or to book Dr. Superson to speak, please contact her at **Camille@DrCamilleSuperson.com**.

www.ingramcontent.com/pod-product-compliance
Lightning Source LLC
Chambersburg PA
CBHW080606270326
41928CB00016B/2945